on
thriving

HARNESSING JOY THROUGH LIFE'S GREAT LABORS

Brandi Sellerz-Jackson

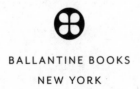

BALLANTINE BOOKS

NEW YORK

On Thriving is a work of nonfiction. Some names and identifying details have been changed.

Published in the United States by Ballantine Books, an imprint of Random House, a division of Penguin Random House LLC, New York.

BALLANTINE BOOKS & colophon are registered trademarks of Penguin Random House LLC.

LIBRARY OF CONGRESS CATALOGING-IN-PUBLICATION DATA
Names: Sellerz-Jackson, Brandi, author.
Title: On thriving : harnessing joy through life's great labors / Brandi Sellerz-Jackson.
Description: First edition. | New York : Ballantine Group, [2024]
Identifiers: LCCN 2023026709 (print) | LCCN 2023026710 (ebook) | ISBN 9780593496671 (hardcover) | ISBN 9780593496688 (ebook)
Subjects: LCSH: Medicine and psychology. | Grief. | Community life.
Classification: LCC R726.5 .S476 2024 (print) | LCC R726.5 (ebook) | DDC 610.1/9—dc23/eng/20230724
LC record available at https://lccn.loc.gov/2023026709
LC ebook record available at https://lccn.loc.gov/2023026710

Printed in the United States of America on acid-free paper

randomhousebooks.com

2 4 6 8 9 7 5 3 1

First Edition

Illustrations by Deun Ivory ART, LLC

Book design by Caroline Cunningham

To Sally, who tilled

Alma, the rebellious thriver

Juril, who remained a constant home

Kimberly, the adventurer

CONTENTS

PART THREE

The Grieving Room

PART FOUR

Thriving While Othered

INTRODUCTION

· ·

When I was a little girl, my mother had a song that she would sing whenever it rained. According to her, the church's old folks would sing it, welcoming the clouds' sweet salve. I imagined the rain baptizing the flowers and blessing the hearts that had harvested them. As my mother sang, I would daydream of the rain's droplets softly kissing the grass that I played on with my cousins in the hot summer sun of Alabama. Our clothing's grass stains would sanctify us and set us apart when we first emerged from indoor comfort to outdoor adventure. I'd imagine the rain sinking deep below the surface, watering the roots, whispering "Grow." The surrounding trees, whose branches would swing low, made it easier for me to climb within them. Their roots, intertwined beneath the surface, held the story of those who came before us. These trees had more than likely seen so very much. I'd imagine the secrets told behind their backs, the kisses exchanged between lovers, and the umbrellalike shelter provided as the rain fell.

Earthworms would make their way aboveground, offering

their uninvited hello. As I sat at my mother's feet, allowing her words to wash away the childlike fear that may have arisen regarding the storm ahead, I would close my eyes and listen to the rain as it fell. The initial pitter-patter and rhythmic salutations were tolerable. It felt like home. However, the sudden thunder and the ebb and flow from the familiar to the unpredictability of the unknown would cause fear to make its grand appearance within my little body. It was the feeling of being so small and helpless, a sensation felt many times at such a young age. This feeling I experienced as a child happens to most of us at some point, when life seems to be out of our control, when the storms threaten our roots. We feel small as life presents itself in all of its terrifying largeness.

Amid nature's chaos, the sound of the rain mixed with my mother's voice called forth a symphony of calm in an otherwise chaotic world. The thunder would clap; my little shoulders would jump. I didn't feel brave. Her song would cause a welcome distraction from my imagination of giants wrestling above. I continued listening to her voice as the rain fell harder upon the roof of our home and knocked against our windows. In that moment, my mother's voice and the steady drumming of rain calmed me.

The lightning bellowed. I remember thinking that, indeed, the sound of thunder was the direct replica of the voice of God, commanding all to stand at attention and in awe. Thunder was the glare that a mother gave during church service, commanding her child to sit up and acknowledge as the preacher delivered their sermon. The thunder was the spoken yet unspoken command to be alert and the directive to act as if you had some damn home trainin'. As the rain fell, I felt a sense of renewal and fear. The rain represented all things clean and the washing away of yesterday. The thunder felt scary and holy at the same time—as our own inner storms often do. I continued to sit, glued to my mother's voice, calling forth the nurturing spirit of the rain for me. Oh, how its presence would call forth nature's growth.

Decades later, on a crisp, wet January morning in 2018, I would find myself standing beneath the rain's guidance, palms open, requesting that just as nature experienced her renewal, I would too. I'd miscarried for the second time. As the spring rain poured outside my home, I recalled the days of my youth sitting at my mother's feet. I ventured out into my front yard and allowed the shower to wash over me. I wasn't sure if the rain could heal my broken heart or if it had the power to cleanse my grief. However, I knew what it could do for the daffodils, the California succulents upon my doorstep, and the sun-scorched grass that needed its care. I, too, was depleted, bare, and dry. I also needed watering, and so here I was.

Hey there, my name is Brandi. I am a birth and postpartum doula who became what I call a Life Doula. This means I have the privilege of supporting people as they journey through this life adventure. We are all giving birth to something. Conceiving a new reality. Laboring through our days as we attempt to capture our joy and hold it close. A doula is quite literally a person that guides and supports people through various life transitions, be it literal birth, postpartum, or death, or a figurative rebirth of oneself into our next path. I help people as they learn to capture said joy, transition through the various rooms of life, and cultivate their highest selves. Over the years, I've worked with many clients, and what has remained true is that we all, no matter the room of life we find ourselves in, want to go from simply surviving to thriving. But it takes work to get there—work we'll do together here to get you to more joy, to a life that thrives.

What's the difference between surviving and thriving? Survival is instinctual. We all want to live. It's in our bones to reach for the sun and oxygen to fill us with life. But thriving is different. It *feels* different. Thriving is the intentional gathering of all things possible and creating the best-case scenario for growth. It looks like using what you have and fearlessly creating more. It's asking yourself "What do I need for the present journey and the road ahead?" Thriving is a rebellious middle finger to the expectation (societal or internal) that we must only exist, sacrificing our experience here on earth. Simply put, I describe thriving as our will to live and breathe and taste life fully, savoring it on our tongue, leaving us full in our belly. My hope is that, with the stories and lessons nestled in this book, you find ways to thrive in the spaces of discomfort. That's been my life's journey.

As a Life Doula, I've witnessed four great labors that we all must move through. Sure, there are likely more, but these four come up again and again across age, background, economic status, and all walks of life. These four great labors of our lives push us to our superpower of vulnerability and her not-so-distant cousin, solidity. These two are often revealed only as we traverse these great labors. However, we can sometimes get stuck in the struggle of it all if we get into a pattern of only weathering life's storms, as they pass over us, instead of giving ourselves precisely what we need as we birth ourselves through to the other side.

Okay, I know you are probably wondering what these four great labors are. First, there is the labor of our relationships. Whether familial, platonic, or romantic, I've learned that relationships can be our most extraordinary hardship or teacher. And when we've yet to really unravel how intimacy and our unhealed wounds play a part in our relationships, we risk not experiencing the freedom of a healthy relationship with ourselves or those around us.

The second great labor concerns our mental health. Understanding our mind and the power of our self-belief is half the battle. We find ourselves in ruts, searching for peace of mind. And while there are modalities to cultivate our mental health (many of which we will discuss in this book), the real work begins with the simple acknowledgment that sometimes we all need support, compassion, and a little bit more, and that there is no shame in that.

The third great labor is dealing with grief and loss. Death is the great uniter. We all get a turn in the laborious work of grief and loss. None of us are exempt from this work. And the question is, "How does one continue after experiencing the breathtaking shift of such labor?" How do we carry on in this world while mourning the departure of what was into another? There is a way, and we will talk through it together.

And finally, the fourth great labor is contending with the title of being othered. Being a member of the marginalized and dealing with the potential weathering that comes with it can leave you feeling depleted and worn. However, despite the beautiful skin we are wrapped in, gender, sexual orientation, or the body that houses the essence and beauty of who you are, *you* are worthy of divine bliss, and defiant freedom. You are worthy of taking up space and taking in love. When we truly embrace this truth despite the world we live in, we too can thrive.

We will walk through each of these laboring rooms of our lives to finally get off the birthing table, sweaty and out of breath from just trying to make it to the next day, beyond the subsequent frustration or discomfort, and move into a thriving life that is wholly ours.

Within the book, I break down each section into those four great labors of our lives, as, for the most part, the vast majority of us will get a turn to occupy each of these spaces. As a woman who has more than forty-five plants scattered across my home and has spent almost a decade in a (mostly) loving, ever-evolving relationship with the wisdom of plants, I use plant symbolism throughout the book as a visual point of reference and cultivator of self-curiosity and checking in. Although I am not a plant expert, I have found that plants serve as an excellent example of a living thing reaching for life itself and gathering (even demanding) what it needs to thrive and grow.

We will visit the room of relationships to unearth our partnership with ourselves and those around us. We will dig into the weeds of our wounds, egos, and the deep desire for connection that have long been hindered. During this time, we will land at a place of sanctuary and self-awareness. We will visit the room of our mental health. We will excavate and dig into our trauma responses and triggers, calloused areas that may have felt too overwhelming to see in the past. We will notice the room of loss, unearthing the process of dormancy and the need for cultivation within "the shit" of grief, landing at a gentle awareness of where to place our feelings after loss that is in deep self-compassion, understanding that the heartache we feel after such loss is just love looking for a place to heal. We will talk through the space of being "othered," be it due to economic status, race, gender identity, ability, or any of the other ways society others us. This othering can feel like the banishing of our bodies, cast out without acceptance or acknowledgment. We will dig through history and how it has added to our othering, our depletion, and the ways of thinking that have found their home within ourselves. In this section, we will reclaim our rest and ourselves while finding our true north. Each chapter offers a set of journal prompts and questions for you to discover and revisit when ready. In this digging, I will guide you toward arriving at a place of knowing safety as your own, even post-trauma.

. . . .

After those two miscarriages, I would blessedly go on to conceive once more and carry to term. The birth of my second child, Jedi, was hard. Actually, hard is an understatement. It was agonizing, brutal, yet somehow, someway, beautiful. It was around nine in the morning when my water broke. I had just gotten out of the shower and begun putting on my underwear when I felt a warm trickle run down my leg and onto the hardwood floor. At first, I thought, "Am I peeing on myself?" Which felt normal, for the record. Like many, my pregnancy was filled with missed bathroom opportunities and failed attempts to make it to the toilet in time. Yes, I peed when I sneezed, and what of it? My water didn't break like in the movies. There was no massive gush, triggering the pandemonium of labor and a mad dash to the hospital or a phone call to the midwife. It was slow and easy, a lazy riverlike trickle, signaling that Jedi was on his way.

I yelled for my husband, Jon, so that he, too, could analyze what was popping in the champagne room. The more I moved, the more water made its exit. It was time, or so I thought, but I still had errands to run. I took my oldest kid to the dentist, and Jon and I went to the grocery store and then for a neighborhood walk. Once home, I bounced on my birth ball. I did all of this, hoping that my baby would make his way earthside soon. My contractions finally came, but they were irregular and would ebb and flow from ten minutes apart to forty-five minutes and then completely stop. During this waiting period of twelve hours, I binge-watched television, ate spicy food, and napped, all in an effort to usher Jedi along.

Day turned into night, and still nothing. By this time, pregnancy had already taught me the lesson of release and the illusion we have of control. Here I was, learning yet another task.

The miscarriage I suffered before Jedi's conception brought along further emotional upendings. Often, after enduring such a loss, one's following pregnancy can be riddled with anxiety of the unknown, which is also true after any loss. Whether you have experienced a harsh breakup or a divorce, it's completely normal that the fear of venturing into another relationship, although excellent and healthy this go-around, can feel frightening and unsettling.

The truth is this life that we live is much bigger than ourselves, and the inner working thereof is above our pay grade and, no doubt, magic. I had to choose to relinquish control and lean into the celebration of the unknown, confident that I could show up as is, holding gratitude for the uncontrollable and the mystery behind it.

Navigating the unfamiliar doesn't feel safe. And we all are looking for a sense of sanctuary within our bodies and within the world around us. Often, we grasp for this safety by performing our hilarious attempt at controlling all variables, including the people around us. When we attempt to control uncontrollable sources, we exhaust ourselves and our energy. In this book, I will share the bizarre beauty of letting go and what it feels like to finally embrace life's messy and uncontrollable moments.

As the hours passed during my early labor with Jedi, it became abundantly clear that once again I wasn't controlling anything. It wasn't until midnight that our then family of three loaded up our car, called our birth gang, and made our way to the hospital. Of course, when I arrived, they checked me and announced that I was only 2–3 centimeters dilated, at which my heart sank deep within my stomach. If you are not familiar with this number's insignificance, allow me to break it down in simpler terms: When a pregnant person is 2–3 centimeters, there is still a long road ahead before baby makes its appearance. Within this moment of frustration, there appeared yet another lesson. Although there was much work to be done and the goal seemed so far away, things were still happening. Progress was being made even within what felt like stagnation. Because my water had broken, the hospital admitted me and took us to our birthing room.

Jon prepared our space. He had packed our most treasured things from home, including one of our favorite salt lamps. We even broke the hospital's rules and burned one of our favorite candles. Miles Davis played on our phones as I performed more bouncing on the birthing ball. Eventually, around four o'clock, we fell asleep in hopes of meeting baby by morning light.

The sun rose with no baby in sight, just hospital breakfast and more bouncing. I stared at the clock, watching and waiting. I would be the first person in the history of *ever* to be pregnant *forever*. I was convinced that this baby of mine had dug his heels down deep into my uterus and was staging a protest. Eventually, my friends would cover the hospital room's clocks, detouring my attention away from all sense of time and distracting me from traveling down the rabbit hole of Google. My hyperfocus on the clock and my progression checklist were not my friends. It hindered me, preventing me from being present—the more I focused on the clock, the less I paid attention to my breath, to connecting with my baby, and most important, to where I was landing physically and emotionally with all of this. Which is something many of us do. We watch the clock and compare as our manifested hopes progress. We hold our breath as if this holding will bring our dreams forward faster. Spoiler alert: It does not.

Watching the clock is a distraction from the present. We put internal pressure on ourselves to achieve more success instead of merely showing up as is and fully ourselves. Sometimes the clock is external. If not careful, we become moved and influenced by those around us regarding what's deemed an accomplishment and compare ourselves to others. We forget that our journey and successes are personal and relative. When we begin to remove the clock of our mind, letting go of timelines and unrealistic goals for our internal clock, that's when we start to grow.

For example, have you ever run into a friend in the grocery store, and they ask, "How are things going? What have you been up to?" This innocent question can provoke immediate anxiety for doing and being more. We can begin to list what we are "doing" and accomplishing. This performing is done so the person on the other end knows we are on schedule with "the clock" of our lives. Imagine, if when we were asked this question, that we were instead to take a breath, cover the clock of our mind, and respond with how we are growing and the lessons we are currently learning. This response takes away the power of not-enoughness and the need to validate one's worth by a timetable. Whether you are running a Fortune 500 company, launching your passion project, or potty training while maintaining your sanity, we all feel pressure to perform and watch the clock of our achievements. I would encourage you to ignore the clock and instead be present, as this is where our expansion for joy and thriving takes shape.

We walked around the hospital, and eventually my contractions kicked into high gear. My conversations started to shorten as my contractions became more intense. I went inward, focusing on my breath, and reminded myself that every contraction was bringing me closer to seeing my baby. I was in transition, which is by far the most challenging part of labor.

I often share that transition is when heaven and earth meet, and if you could pack your bags and vacate the premises, you would. I like to refer to transition as "the door." Like our life's journey, the door can be seen as a crossroads, a turning point. It is the deciding factor to either sink or swim. Within this sacred moment, the birthing person and their baby are the only ones who can walk through the door, as it is their journey.

Labor's transition has been known to bring up any and everything below the surface. For example, if there is childhood trauma, expect this to come up by looking for the need to control the birthing process. Within labor, a birthing person who has experienced such trauma may find themselves searching for stability and the "adults" in the room—all of this is done to locate and feel safe. Childbirth is a highly vulnerable time. As a birth guide, I share with families that doulas are not epidurals. We are not magic, and when reaching "the door" of transition, there will be no amount of pixie dust, palo santo, or kind words that will get them through it, only their sheer grit, breath, and the teacher within, which we have been cultivating up until that point. Sages have correlated this transition moment during labor to pregnant people leaving their bodies to retrieve their babies' souls.

Labor transition is a hallowed place, and I hadn't felt the hallelujah of it all within my birth. The hallelujah was on the other side of my pain. The same is true for you too. Our labors within this life meet transition within the most challenging moments. Moments when our spirit and body are sometimes being pushed to their limits. Within these challenging moments, the kind that cause you to doubt your fortitude, strength, and yourself, is the moment one must actively choose to make friends with the discomfort. This is how you emerge on the other side, sitting within the exhaustion and power of your most arduous life work.

I wanted the pain and the uncertainty to end. The lack of stability and the unknown within this experience felt vastly familiar and reminiscent of my early childhood. I didn't feel I could keep going. By this point, nature had pushed my body to the brink.

My hips widened and cracked, blossoming life itself through. The time for harvest was near, and I knew it to be true. A wise friend of mine had prepared me pre-labor with the sage advice, "When you get to the point of wanting to quit, and when your doubt begins to overpower truth, you are almost there. Keep going. Your baby is on the other side of your breath." My breath became shallow, reflecting the fear and past trauma experienced. I called for my mother, who had passed on. I wanted her near. I desired to nestle close to her as if I were a babe myself. Tears fell as I called out for her and any other source of comfort. I had made it to the point that I never thought I could. As pain made its way through my body, I was reminded that this pain wasn't a bad thing; instead, it was the portal.

Each contraction was a step forward. This pain would bring me closer to my son. These moments I refer to as "the waves." While you are navigating hard life moments, I ask that you imagine these moments as incoming tides. And know that you possess the choice to either fight against them or to surrender to their power, trusting that the tide will not break you—that it will carry you through. The wave is your friend, as is the discomfort. It is all a bridge to your joy. During childbirth, I was reminded that I could thrive within the wildness, pain, and intensity of my experience. One moment at a time. One breath at a time.

Birth is wild. Primal. Ancestral and ancient. It's unapologetically carefree and gives zero fucks, like many of the uncontrollable events life throws our way. Birth is also a teacher, guiding the lucky participant through lessons from their past and along the winding road ahead. During labor, I remember feeling connected to something more profound than what could be seen or touched. I felt my mother and grandmother and her mother before. I felt the holiness of childbirth and all of its sweetness— the deep-rooted feeling of strength embodied within my bones.

Much like anything containing a seed, I had grown an offspring—
a human. For nine months, I had waited patiently to meet my
labor of love. Now the moment was at hand.

As mentioned, birth can be a teacher. However, this teacher
lives inside each and every one of us. And during our time together, I will share not only how you can access this teacher, but
also how in many ways you *are* the teacher. And if we listen
closely, we all can hear them instructing us through. Our inner
teacher will always point us to our highest truth and keep us on
the pathway of opportunity for growth. Throughout our time together, I will reference your inner teacher so that you can better
identify, recognize, and connect to its voice when it speaks. Your
teacher may be your breath and the attunement thereof. Your
teacher may be the inner nudge to advocate for yourself within
a space where advocacy is not present. It is the inner voice that
prioritizes both your emotional and mental safety. Your teacher
may be the pause before you agree and say yes. Your teacher
should feel reminiscent of home and a warm hug. The internal
pat on the back that reminds you that you are powerful enough
to keep moving forward. I hope that with this book you will
begin to trust your intuition, your body, and the teacher within—
that you will realize you already have everything you need to
thrive.

The lessons I learned during Jedi's delivery were that of letting go, releasing, and more explicitly thriving within any space
inhabited (even the tough ones). Yes, I wanted to survive Jedi's
birth, a feat that was not guaranteed to me statistically as a Black
woman due to our country's medical system. However, I wanted
to thrive within it as well. I wanted to experience bliss within the
uncontrollable and call it friend. My blissful moment wouldn't

come until after I birthed Jedi. Feeling the release rush within myself and finally holding my child was otherworldly. I felt powerful, not merely because of the way I chose to birth, but because I navigated my pregnancy with intention, fortitude, and, more specifically, with autonomy. I had leaned into the anxiety around my pregnancy after loss, taking back my power while conquering fear and the illusion of control. I had even opted to sink deep into the discomfort and birth my vision on my terms, and I hope that you will do the same.

Often, I compare our thriving to that of plant life. After all, we humans aren't that different from plants in our need for water and sunshine. We both navigate and actively search for the most hospitable spaces to live and grow. We forage our way through areas of gratitude, triumph, happiness, joy, or denser emotions, such as loss, grief, and disappointment. What would happen if, despite the headspace we're in, we gleaned a few lessons from nature and began to nurture our whole selves, asking the question "What do I need in this present condition to thrive?"

I have borne witness to many who emerge with more clarity, awareness of self, and practical ways of personal sustainability by asking this question of themselves, like my client Susan, who was a parent of a little one in the NICU. She began feeling overwhelmed in caring for herself and her postpartum body and making daily trips to care for her baby. She grieved for the pregnancy and birth for which she had hoped. I had so much admiration for this mother's strength and wisdom to reach out for support.

During our first session together, I asked her the question, "What do you need within this moment?" She expressed that she had to take a moment to ask herself this simple question because she had not had the time to even consider this. I simplified it even more for her: "Do you need water? Do you need to take a shower? Do you need to cry?" She immediately began to list the first thing she needed and then the second. First, she expressed that she needed a nap. She hadn't slept well for a while. This question propelled her on the journey of checking in with herself so that she could continue to show up for her child and thrive.

She and I worked together for the duration that her little one was in the NICU. She checked in with herself during that time and asked that formerly unfamiliar question. This newly introduced ritual eventually became second nature. This question would span beyond childbirth, pregnancy, and what she was currently navigating. The practice of asking herself this question, a simple human question, was one that she would carry within her thriving and sustainability toolbox forever.

In my work as a birth and postpartum guide, I have had the honor of supporting and doulaing people through the various spaces of pregnancy and childbirth. I began this work after the birth of Jedi. After experiencing loss, miscarriage, and postpartum isolation, my heart grew for those attempting to find the joy, the celebration, and the opportunity for expansion not only during childbirth but also in the ordinary day-to-day. As I said earlier, we are all giving birth to something. My offering to you as you read this book is simple: Allow all of the parts—all your emotions—to be a catalyst for your joy. For me, grief was the starter. I birthed my blog, *Not So Private Parts,* after experiencing pregnancy loss. I saw a need for a safe space for those who had encountered such emotional upheaval and disappointment, so I created one. The same is true for Moms in Color, an organization I co-founded, centering Black motherhood, joy, and community. In that case, frustration was the starter. I was actively searching for a path to self-celebration and a safe space for expression. In my experience, the way to joy and healing is and will always be *through*. Since then, I have created a pathway of following one's highest bliss through discovery and intentional digging and unearthing, as this curiosity is how we find nuggets of truth and gold buried beneath our foundation.

I should probably share now that there is no such thing as an arrival at thriving, but rather a constant journey of unpacking and packing what you need for the adventure ahead. Like my labor story and stories of the birthing people whom I have had the privilege of guiding, thriving where you are is filled with waiting, summoning, breathing through, and leaning into the discomfort of it all so that you can celebrate the joy and its fruits. It is trusting our path and our body, covering the clocks, making peace, and becoming friends with the relinquishing, a lesson that repeats itself throughout life's great labors. Thriving is leaning into the fear and the uncertainty. It is sitting at the feet of thunder and allowing it to not only teach us but mother us in the stillness. I reflect on those moments as a little girl in the rain, sitting at the feet of my mother, and how as she would sing her song of the rain, I became a little less afraid of the boisterous lightning. I was unaware then, but my mother taught me a valuable lesson on connection and grounding. Her voice felt like a compass directing me toward my North Star of self-awareness. As long as I could lead my attention back to her voice, to the one thing that was still, the one thing that was quiet and sure, then I would be okay. At that moment, she would meet me there, inside the fear, reaffirming that I could be both afraid and brave, still and growing, within that very moment. The lesson taught by the rain, my mother, and me, established a beautiful foundation of growing despite fear and the uncontrollable. As I listened to my mother's voice, she taught me the lesson of thriving in whatever space I inhabited.

Thriving is dancing with yourself, preparing a decadent meal (because that's what you may need), and in my case, being Black AF while centering and cultivating joy as an act of resistance. It's creating rituals and viewing their practice as a tool that enriches us all. After all, our "rich-uals" should constantly enrich us. It's continual watering and caring for self, checking in from moment to moment, between the celebration and exploration, the gathering and the casting away. When it comes to thriving, it's safe to say that one is continually navigating the how-to's and the inner workings of it all. Akin to the childlike exploration that most of us experienced during our youth, one must possess that same curiosity to grow. There are no quick fixes when it comes to our maturation. There is only the tenacity and bravery to root down into the deep dirt of our programming so that we can flourish in tandem with the hope of a bright future ahead.

Dear reader, I hope that you will begin to not only survive but thrive by reading this book. Within its pages, I hope to simplify your self-care practice so that you can tap into the teacher that is birthed within. After you complete this book, I hope you will use it as a gentle reminder and companion for checking in and continuing the ritual of asking yourself, "What is it that I need to thrive within the space that I'm in?" Life is a labor of love. Here are the lessons I've learned along the way. Here's to all the rooms where we catch and allow the light in. May we grow.

Lord, it's gonna rain.
It's gonna rain.
You better get ready and bear this in mind . . .
                                        —OLD SPIRITUAL

· ·

PART ONE

Thriving in Relationship with Oneself and Others

GLADYS AND RICK, ROSE AND GARLIC

Although different, roses and garlic grow well together.
The garlic bulbs repel pests that would otherwise seek out
the rosebud. May we give thanks for dissimilarities,
including the bitter things, for they nurture our growth.

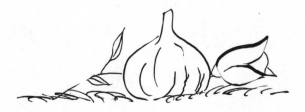

CHAPTER ONE

Lighting the Black Hole

I remember the first time that I touched myself.
Touching the parts that were locked away and unseen . . .
in deep need of repair.
Searching for joy and intimacy.

I would like to tell you that my first time experimenting with
psychedelics was somewhere far away yet so very typical, like
Indio, California, or Joshua Tree, surrounded by nature seques-
tered in a yurt, where my friends and I lit incense as we set our
intentions while partaking in mushrooms going away on our psychedelic trip, wild and free. That we heard and tasted the colors
of the dry and desolate paradise around us, engrossed by just
how high we really were. This ideal and imagined scenario is
how I'd always seen it portrayed in the White sitcoms and movies, granting the lucky participants the permission for complete
and utter exploration that I, a Black woman, had yet to experience. I'd never gone through the typical experimental phase in
my teenage years or early twenties. I didn't frequent my college
town's pub or club shooting tequila shots while noshing on bar
fries and poppers, let alone attend a rave where psychedelics
would more than likely be present. This kind of youthful exploration was not afforded to kids who looked like me. I grew up

knowing that being too unrestricted and too wild could get you locked up, killed, or worst, underage and pregnant.

So instead of experimenting in the desert, there I was in my late thirties in therapy discussing the possibility of incorporating psychedelics into my treatment for generalized anxiety and trauma. I sat in the chair, afraid. I was fearful not of what could happen while on my psychedelic trip, but what and who I would possibly see, and of letting go of control—the letting go being the most terrifying and the most challenging part. Up until this point, I'd held on to as much control as possible. The therapist assured me that I would be okay, while also instructing me to be vulnerable and to simply "go with it." I am convinced that she had no idea the weight of what she was asking. I had always been required to be aware, vigilant, and alert. By the time I was an adult, I had encountered varying traumas, all before the age of thirteen, all of them while also being Black and woman. And now I was being asked to take down the very fortifications that were all designed and constructed to keep me safe.

Before my trip, I tried my hand at what I would see. I was sure that I would have this heartfelt conversation with my mother and heal the wounds inflicted by my father. During my trip, I would talk to all the adults in my life as a child. I tried to grab whatever bit of control that one could seize before going on a trip of this nature. I'd heard all the horror stories of "bad trips," people seeing things that they'd only seen in their worst nightmares. The therapist assured me that I would see only what I needed to see, the parts that trauma had long ago locked away inside a vault, too cautious and too afraid to make their way to the surface. She sat in her armchair, staring across at me, explaining how our brain seals memories away after trauma. And how, hopefully, this session would not only open my mind but allow those closeted memories to present themselves. She said this as if it was a good thing. For someone who had seen what I'd seen growing up, the closet of my subconscious felt like a black hole, frightening, a place that I had yet to explore.

I was fearful because of what I knew of the subconscious and how it presented itself once given permission. It was like the magic eight-ball toy of the '80s. Ask a question, shake it, and stare, waiting for the plaything's all-knowing answer to somehow cause the world to make a little more sense. I dreaded and agonized over entering the black hole of the hidden and unattended wounds of our lives. But the black hole is where we find the origin of ourselves. Our true selves. The parts that knew to run and hide because they were far too ugly or uneasy to be seen. Too fragile. It is this place where we often need to begin. What happens when we discover the mother wound? The wound that continued to birth other injuries in its stead? The poet Rumi says, "The wound is where the light enters you." Although unhealed, perhaps oozing even, our wound is the entry point for all things light to find us and make their home. The acknowledgment of its existence is the beginning of our healing journey.

Music, dance parties, and family gatherings were ever-present during my early childhood. Laughter and shit-talking, stories of yesterday embellished by ego and bravado, bounced off the walls and onto the streets. Grown-ups talked about grown-up business. We children knew our place of playing outside and running back into the house when the streetlights came on. There was always that one relative who lacked a sense of boundaries, placing a slobbery kiss on your cheek and then proceeding to fix their plate, finding their place at their nautical striped folding beach chair. The R&B song "Casanova" would play over the radio, which had also made its way outside. There was joy and a congregation of parents gathered in a circle to show off their children during our dance circle and self-ordained *Soul Train* line. If there was one thing that Black parents in the '80s loved to do, showing off their kids dancing amongst relatives was it. I looked forward to these moments of communion. Within this gathering of trusted family existed safety. Outside its protection, that sense of emotional and physical security would vanish once I returned home.

At our humble home in Bristol, Connecticut, the dancing, music, and joy would cease, and the battering of my mother, Kimberly, by my father, Greg, would begin. My father suffered from addiction, often self-soothing with drugs and alcohol. Pots and pans would fall to the floor, and the sound of thunder clapping would make its presence known, except this time, the giants wrestling were my mother and father. I would try to stop the fights. However, what could I do? At the age of six, I was no match for my father, who was well over six feet tall. Greg struggled with undiagnosed mental illness and the residue of childhood trauma. At times, I would place my body between them in hopes of stopping the war. My six-year-old frame would become sandwiched between the two adults as I hoped that perhaps my bravery would create space for peace. Along with my role as referee, my search for safety had begun. I would search not only for the adults in the room but for the safe spaces, the free spaces, and the spaces where I could feel the autonomy of curiosity that most children my age had naturally set out to discover.

My mother, my little sister, who was only a baby, and I entered a domestic violence shelter as I neared my seventh birthday. We arrived early evening, and the sun had yet to set. I still remember the parking lot and how it presented as a sacrosanct and private place, encircled with tall green bushes blocking the building. No signage marked the establishment to keep those inside of its walls safe. I waited outside the office, where my mother talked with the woman on the other side of the door. My mother was afraid, in her mid-twenties and far away from her childhood home of Sylacauga, Alabama. She'd had me when she was nineteen years old, just a few short years after running away with my father up north. My mother sat inside the enclosed office, sharing her story with the woman providing intake. Much of it, I'm sure she didn't want me to hear. However, I knew as much as a child could understand. I knew that things must have gotten really bad as this was the first time I remembered my mother leaving my father.

That night, the three of us lay snuggled in one queen-sized bed. The warm blankets covered us as we lay in each other's arms, my sister between us. I remember the blackness of the room, with one gleaming nightlight that shone in the corner next to the bedside table. In what felt like the holiest of holy temples, I lay in that bed, feeling for the first time that I could rest and finally exhale the breath that I had been holding.

The next day, I sat huddled around the table with the other kids who lived there. We ate fish sticks with ketchup, all smiling and giggling. The thing that we all had in common was that we had seen more than any child should see. Our mothers had escaped violence toward themselves and toward their children. I remember smiling and laughing with them because they, too, carried a secret. Like me, they used guardedness and being more innovative and quick-witted as tools for survival. We stayed a week or so in the shelter before my mother returned to my father. There was no conversation—just a return. As a child, I was torn. I didn't understand why she would return to my father. Perhaps this is the complex thing about these fortresses that we call home. We long for it even when it leaves us in disorder. My guess is that this time, like times before, my father had promised that he would never _____ again or he would stop _____. That this time would be different, that he was now different, that he had changed during her absence. Whatever his story, she believed him, and back we went. And like many times before, the song and dance would continue. After he would abuse my mother or enter a state of rage, the cops would be called. He would be taken away. He would return. Changed, and yet not. Wash and repeat.

In that same year, our family would eventually move from the small town of Bristol to another small town, Sylacauga. My mother had made her way back to her childhood home, except this time with her two daughters and my father, now her husband.

Sylacauga was different. It was a wild and untamed culture shock in every way imaginable. According to my classmates, I talked funny. I wore my hair funny. More than likely, I also looked funny. My mother would adorn my hair with oversized bows. I had prominent features and full cheeks, into which I had yet to grow. My garments also seemed to run bigger than hoped for against my tiny frame. I had yet to grow into those too. My parents, like many back then, extended the life of their kids' clothing by purchasing everything a size or two too big. In my head, I was a seven-year-old fly girl ripped from the television show *In Living Color*. I hoped to look like a cross between one of their dancers and the teen dream Debbie Gibson.

There was no need for snow boots or snowsuits there in Alabama. The snow somehow knew its boundaries and how far to take its ice-cold grasp even in winter. One would think that my father possessed the same intuition after our southern migration. As a child, I thought that perhaps living so close to my grandmother and family would protect us from his violent episodes. It did not. The abuse would worsen. As a child, I'm not sure why this was. He seemed angrier and on a razor-sharp edge that we all had to tiptoe around, or else hell would erupt. Or maybe I was getting older, and the reality of my childhood being steeped in and surrounded by violence could and would no longer be hidden behind closed doors and violent grown-folk conversations.

HIDING THE KNIVES AND SURVIVAL

While witnessing my father's abuse, I would hide the kitchen knives, hoping that this simple act of being one step ahead would protect the adults in the room. As a child, my thought process was: *If I just hide everything that can cause harm, everyone will be safe.* This protection was for my mother, my sister, myself, and my father. By the age of nine, I'd begun my ritual of hiding sharp objects. Greg had attempted suicide multiple times. And although, as a child, I didn't know the full details of his intentions to end his life, I knew and felt my role of being my father's safe-keeper intuitively, even if that meant protecting him from himself. My ritual of hiding the knives would be the genesis of my taking on the responsibility of being the official adult in the room throughout my life.

I felt the need to protect my mother from the chaos of my father. I also wanted to protect my father from his internal danger. For the record, this search for safety wouldn't end, even after my parents divorced four years later. This time of my life birthed my mother wound. This ritual of hiding all the sharp objects, all the dangerous things, all that could cause harm, was my way of moonlighting as the person in charge of keeping everyone around me safe while also attempting to architect a world that felt safe to me as well.

What rituals did you pick up as a child in order to survive? And are you still using them today? Did you strive for perfection in order to receive love? Were you walking in Dad's shoes hoping that this imitation meant he'd not abandon you? Maybe you simply followed all the rules to keep the peace and still do so until this day when your inner peace is threatened? We all have rituals we've developed from our childhood, rituals that formed while trying to grow a scab over our mother wound. However, we can't really get to the other side, to the good, thriving life, without first recognizing them and analyzing whether they still serve us. For me, the childhood rituals developed in the darker moments of my life stayed with me for decades and seemed to be an armor of protection—keyword "seemed."

During my childhood, there was no room to grow into myself unattached from trauma. There was no time to get to know myself intimately beyond the survival of the day-to-day, between experiencing the almost weekly abuse by my father against my mother and taking on the emotional task of managing my surroundings and the adults within them. Daily fear would suck the very air of any early self-awareness out of the room and out of my grasp. During those years, I was not afraid of the boogey monster; instead, I was both physically and mentally knowledgeable of the screams for help, chairs sliding, and the things that would go bump in the night. The fear experienced was visceral. It would prove impossible to begin to discover who I was or could be while taking on the task of family manager and peacekeeper. This kind of finding takes time and safety. Time developed amid the ease of watching Saturday morning cartoons and enjoying a bowl of cereal, a life where kids can be kids and not adults. My stomach lived in knots as I'd play a game of knife keep-away, tucking the sharp objects beneath my bed, as I was sure it was the one place no one would find them. My childhood was too occupied with loud voices overpowering my own, and my body felt too shared, sandwiched as a barrier between my parents. There was no peace within this self-imposed duty, only constant alertness and vigilance. The ritual of keeping the people around me safe would become my own safe space, though to my detriment. Staying within the lines, making sure to not harm, in word or deed, would become my oath and path until I chose that it was not.

My father would have good moments, tender moments even. He wasn't always mad or raging. And although he suffered from addiction, he wasn't always drunk or high. Sometimes, when my mother would work the early-morning shift, he would get me ready for school in the morning, help me gather my clothes and brush my hair. These moments were so sweet that it was hard to believe that the same hands that pushed me on the playground swing could double as the hands that perpetuated abuse. I learned quickly that people were and could be all things. That they could be both loving and cruel, and that they contained layers upon layers of the unknown draped like coats upon their character.

This unpredictability of humans made me afraid of them. And so I would try my hand at controlling the world around me, pre-empting the humans. I would hide the sharp objects because no one would get hurt if I could eliminate them from the equation. I would try my hand at forecasting, imagining the outcome and what I would do if things went awry. I would imagine all the what-ifs, and whether my mother would need the sharp objects I had hidden. I had already determined that I wouldn't unknowingly contribute to a situation where my mother could die by my father's hand. I imagined myself stepping in and saving the day like the superheroes I saw on television. I imagined running to my bed, swiftly grabbing a knife from underneath, and with sleight of hand, passing it to my mother for her protection.

CHILDHOOD AND OUR MOTHER WOUND

We all have the choice to put aside the ways our childhood rituals worked to protect us. By continuing these rituals we never get the chance to explore who we are outside of our survival tactics. Sure, we have our good days. Days when it seems the residue of our childhood barely touches our current and future selves. And then, suddenly, we are triggered and revert back to unhealthy patterns. I also know that my childhood may have held a different level of trauma than yours, but we are all shaped by our childhood, and it's the room we must unpack first to thrive as adults in this crazy world.

Why childhood? Why begin here? Because here lies the genesis of our wounds. And while my scars may look and feel different from yours, they are all worthy of being fully seen and healed. Some people may find it futile to venture into the past. After all, we can't change it. However, remember the wound. Remember the light.

Many don't desire to journey back into the forgotten spaces of childhood because we've been unintentionally taught not to respect the humanity and validity of children's experiences. As a child, were your feelings validated? Or did you hear "It wasn't that bad" or "You survived, didn't you?" If you were encouraged to move on quickly as a child or to simply "get over it," there's a high probability that it is difficult for you to hold space for your childhood, fully feeling the depths of what you experienced. One eventually develops a numbed callus over the entire experience. We adopt the notion that it no longer matters, and therefore why visit this abandoned room? So we never call ourselves back into our childhood memories, and there the initial wound stays neglected, hurt, traumatized, and ultimately unhealed. If we don't journey back to its conception, this wound continues to bleed and seep into the present.

REVISITING AS A BALM

I, too, for so long refused to visit the abandoned land of childhood. There it lay desolate, devoid of breath and air. I would minimize my experience altogether by the standard of "Well, no one died." I would silence the little voice that would scream out in unrecognized fear. It wasn't until my late thirties that I spoke to my grandmother over the phone regarding my experience. It was her eighty-first birthday. I shared with her the joys of writing this book and how establishing home became a common theme throughout. I conveyed to her my gratitude for her home and how it always felt like a sanctuary, surrounding and protecting me. And as I shared with my grandmother that her home was the place where I could go and feel . . . she finished my sentence and said, "safe." She said, "My home was where you could come and just sleep . . . without fear." And in that sacred moment, for the first time, I knew and felt that what I had seen and regarded as a child was real. The constant state of fear and perpetual anxiety lived not only in my head, was frozen not only in time but in truth. As an adult, remembering childhood can feel like the daunting task of reassembling all the unassembled and confusing pieces. Hearing my grandmother speak of the disparity and frightening understanding of my childhood validated that it was true. The fear of loud noises and the constant need to hold it together was also true.

Through my conversation with my grandmother, I learned

that we can visit our childhood through an intentional conversation with family and friends who may have witnessed our experience (however, making sure that this is family that feels safe is vital). These secure conversations provide support and will help to validate your knowledge of what happened and your wound. It may also show an additional perspective, enabling you to revisit from multiple vantage points. Maybe you don't know or have anyone within your family who can validate your experience with the same warmth and honesty I received from my grandmother. If this is you, I would like to serve as an assurance for you, as my grandmother did for me, and offer these words to you: *It happened. It was real. It does not just live in your head, nor is it fiction.* I want you to know that whether you have someone who can validate your experience or not, what happened to you matters. It mattered then, and it matters now.

When I decided to take the journey into my childhood, I considered the following and would suggest you do so as stepping stones forward:

We must set intentions before unearthing and delving into our childhood. Our intentions act as a sort of North Star for when things get a bit challenging, so we keep sight of why we are here doing this work together. (And no, you are not alone on this journey. We are all right there with you. Digging.) Setting intentions can look like this: "I want to sort through the black hole of childhood because I want to discover why I never quite feel safe, even where there is no threat of danger." You may want to dig through your childhood because no matter your success, you need more. It may be another reason or a culmination of reasons. Knowing your why and setting your intention will keep you steady and focused on the path forward, on the path inward. It will also

serve as protection against unnecessary reintroduced trauma.
A bit of forewarning when beginning on this path: It is super
easy to become entrenched in past trauma. If you are not
careful, the work can start to do the opposite of the intent,
reopening the wound instead of healing it. There is a difference between unearthing trauma for the sake of healing and
suturing, and unearthing just to leave it sitting there out in
the open. Intentions will help you distinguish between the
two. Knowing why will support your discernment in asking
whether this is helpful and healing, or is in direct opposition
to your recovery.

**Acknowledge fear that may be present when you take
the plunge into the deep and murky waters of childhood.**
Is there fear? What are you afraid of? I was scared of what
I would discover to be an accurate depiction. As much as I
deeply desired validation that my experience was real, there
was a part of me that wanted to continue to believe that it
wasn't as bad as I remembered and that I could chalk up my
terrifying experience to my childhood stature and the grown-
ups being so very big and scary. Hearing from my grandmother that it was as terrible as I remember would bring
grief that I would eventually have to mourn and unpack.
Who wants that? So, I get it. Allowing our childhood memories to stay tucked away in a distant past left in dicey remembrance feels more manageable. The fear of digging deep and
unearthing calls for certain bravery. However, I want you to
know that you are worthy of learning more about why you
are the way you are and why you are here in this place now,
asking why.

Who is to blame? I discovered that the further I delved
into my childhood, the more I wanted to blame. I wanted
someone to be at fault for everything I experienced and the

reason I was currently sitting in the therapist's office while they administered psychedelics. I wanted to punish someone, anyone, with blame. And truthfully, the easy target would have been my father. He was the one who created trauma upon trauma, right? However, when I began to go down that road, I discovered that if I blamed him, then I would have to blame the one who caused him to become the person I knew, and then the person who caused that trauma, and the person before that, until I ran out of names or faces that I knew. And believe me when I say that's where our work begins when delving into childhood—allowing ourselves to take honest stock of who we subconsciously blame among the adults who made the adults who made the adults who made us. Because when we do this as far back as we can until we touch slavery, the Holocaust, sexual abuse, or secrets kept for as long as they could be saved like heirlooms passed down, we see that the adults were people who suffered their own trauma and they made people with this unhealed trauma who then made us. And in that place, that's where we can find compassion. And wow, let's just say compassion is what you will need along this thriving journey— a great deal of it.

The world
Your family
Your friends
They may and will all need you
But most importantly,
You need you.

Our childhood, although distant, is not far removed from the core of who we are now. Our hopes, fears, and monsters under the bed remain, just in a different form. The more I remembered little girl Brandi, the more I could hold space and understand my present self. I became more aware of her and in deeper relationship with her.

SELF-INTIMACY

The relationship we have with ourself is the most important relationship we will ever have. It's why we must excavate and nurture every part of the journey, from childhood to present day. It is our first relationship birthed from the moment we enter this world. And while many may think that our parents and adult caretakers are our first relationship, they are not. They are our first external relationship. My relationship with myself and the idea of self-intimacy wouldn't arrive until well within adulthood. I define self-intimacy as a deep knowledge of oneself. Similar to our external relationships, it is consistent learning as we continuously evolve, and it is a practice, not a destination. I define it as knowing, or at least being willing to learn, ourself in every developmental phase. It's knowing and deciphering our voice as our own apart from others and those around us, finding it at its youthful genesis and unearthing it even when it is buried deep within the silt. Audre Lorde said, "If I didn't define myself for myself, I would be crunched into other people's fantasies for me and eaten alive." It is so for those who never fully become self-aware, for those who never become intimate with themselves.

And it's so easy to do, to bypass the relationship that means the most, because everyone needs us. Our jobs, family, friends, and so we ourselves often prioritize all of these external contracts above the one we have with ourself. When we opt out of taking the journey of knowing who we are at our core, of uncovering and healing old wounds, we risk falling into roles that we were never meant to play, all to be consumed by those who prey (unknowingly and knowingly) on our unawareness.

I spent so much of my twenties searching, still afraid of people and their potential for harm, that I would have a tough time simply accepting the good things finding their way to my life. What seemed like a kind friend immediately drove me to become guarded, alert, and cautious. "Why would they want to be friends with me? They'll soon find out I'm not as cool as they think I am. They will quickly discover that I'm not as warm or kind or" (insert all the lies we tell ourselves about ourselves).

It was hard to accept. And so, this was my beginning.

HEALING THE WOUND

Why did I try psychedelics? Because before this work, I was a long way off from truly practicing self-intimacy. Sure, I'd been working professionally as a doula for some time. Still, in doing so, it was easy to disappear within the lives of my clients instead of my own, and the familiarity of being woken in the middle of the night to tend to those who needed my aid. I'd been a doula long before training or certification. There was no ritual to pass through or consent given that I even wanted to do this work. I was a child and also a doula before I knew what that was. This is why psychedelics felt like the path for me. Because I felt like a stranger living in this body. A houseguest, timidly accepting packages for perhaps my neighbor and not myself. Been there? For once in my life, I wanted to begin. I wanted to visit the black hole, as fear-inducing as it seemed, and excavate it, the childhood traumas and the rituals born out of them. I craved the simple yet revolutionary act of embodying this life, not as a sitter watching and waiting for the moment the rightful lessor asks for its return, but as my own.

And so there I was, not in Joshua Tree, but in a therapist's office, waiting, as the nurse administered the first dose of Ketamine, a psychedelic used initially in anesthesia but now used in this alternative therapy practice called Ketamine Assisted Therapy. Almost immediately, the world went from side tables and reclining chairs to pitch black, surrounded by sprinkles of silver dust and what seemed to be constellations. I looked around as I lay suspended within the black walls of the universe, hovering above nothingness. I was horizontal within the black of space, and there I noticed this statue that my fingers clutched for dear life, almost as if this monument was the very thing keeping me from falling to my death within the trip. I clung to the statue as we both lay arrested. As I looked at the bust, I saw it was identical to me. I mean, it looked exactly like me. I hung on to the statue, hands folded around it, and then arms, all to keep from falling. I couldn't see beneath me, as the ground below was pitch black.

But then I remembered the therapist's instructions before the session: "If you are holding on to something, let go." And so I did. I let go. I let go and began to fall and fall and fall some more. Soon to discover that there was no ground beneath me, just more and more opportunity to fall. I tumbled, and then I fell, and my body felt weightless, blowing through the macrocosm. I continued to fall until, eventually, the falling felt like flying.

THE THREE QUESTIONS

As I was falling, I felt both nowhere and everywhere. I felt as though I was a part of everything and absolutely nothing. I felt infinite as if my body were made of a billion speckles of light being dispersed. I felt a kinship with the stars, as I had with my cousins or the kids I met briefly in the shelter. I, too, knew their secrets. The stars whispered, "You are safe, and all is okay." I trusted them. And at that moment, I instinctively asked myself three questions . . .

Who am I?

Where am I?

How long have I been here?

Who am I? I felt so intimately connected to this strange new world around me during my trip that I wasn't quite sure who I was. I was so connected to the grandness of the stars and the sun that I felt detached from who I had known myself to be, small, unsafe, and often unimportant. *Where am I?* I didn't know. I had never been here before. I had never touched this place where I could free-fall as effortlessly as though I were walking. *How long have I been here?* It felt like I'd been there forever. So much so that I began to wonder if I would ever return and if it were a possibility that I would exist here forever. Eventually, I returned to where I was before, in the cushioned seat, across from my guide.

My experience with psychedelics was the moment that I began to see myself more clearly. I awakened from my trip, piecing together all the parts of what I saw. The black vastness of the sky and how the stars within its greatness shone around me and bore witness as I first clung to the statue but eventually found the courage to let go. And because I let go of the figure and began falling, although fearful of crashing, it felt as though these same stars held me close, cheering me on. Proud of me even. I now saw that I am just as brilliant as those stars shining despite the darkness and that I could let go of all the antiquated tools that no longer served a purpose within my present adult self. We are so much larger than the statues we erect to keep us safe.

DISCOVERING THE WOUND

We humans are as vast as the sky. You are not what you've relied on to survive. Who we are is so much more resounding than the fortresses of survival we've built up around us. Before this, I had embarked on the road of healing childhood and present wounds. However, this would be the first time I would *know the origin* of the damage (that mother wound) and how I could begin to heal by getting to know the little girl.

Picture it this way: The wound is everything aboveground. The origin is the roots. Through my psychedelic trip, I could finally see the source and unlock the core memories beyond the wound's surface. For example: Hiding knives as a child to keep those around me safe was a core wound. However, I discovered through my trip that hiding knives wasn't the end of the story, but a tool I adopted to survive. This deeper understanding beyond the wound was the origin. In this space, because I was able to see the lifelessness of the statue and how I clung to it as a child clinging to its parent, I was able to see for the first time my innate childlike desire and lack of protection. For the first time, I saw this desire in a tangible form. I clung to it, hoping that I would stay safe if I did everything right to keep everything in order. I wasn't entirely aware of one exact event that tilted the microcosm of my universe. Still, I knew at that moment, as I adhered like a child to what would keep me from falling, that the roots of these scars flowed deep and way past the present moment, far into a land forgotten, into childhood.

Before we can ask how to thrive within our relationships or any other space, we must first nurture our relationship with ourself and learn to thrive within it. We become deeply intimate with our selfhood, asking the question I asked during my psychedelic trip, "Who am I?" For so long, I had claimed the title of protector and manager. I managed the adults around me as a child, keeping them safe. My nervous system as a child lived in a constant state of activation. And because of this, I never felt safe. Who was I? I was unsafe, and because of this, I was broken, looking and craving for someone to fix me. One of the things that stuck out for me on my trip was the statue. This statue was my face chiseled in stone. I remember clinging to that face, marveling and questioning why there was a statue in space, let alone why it looked like me. It wasn't until I let go that I realized what it represented within my trip and in my life.

Before I began this work, I was an overperformer. I thrived on meeting deadlines and exceeding expectations. I found great fulfillment in "winging it." If you had asked me what my superpower was before I set out on my psychedelic trip, I would have answered without hesitation, "I know how to go with the flow. I am adaptable." And while, sure, being flexible is an important quality to possess, I discovered that my gravitational pull to flying by the seat of my pants was rooted in my survival tools.

Because I was constantly on high alert as a child, there was no time to think about my next step intentionally. It was all reactive. I hear a loud noise, I react to stay safe. Parents are fighting, I react to maintain peace. I had to constantly acclimate to the moves of the adults in the room, and I became great at it.

As an adult, I would avoid planning at all costs and call it creative freedom. My brain had been hard-wired to stay alert to be great at springing to my feet, jabbing and moving like a heavyweight champion. The idea of planning or moving purposefully, well, I simply didn't know how. It wasn't until I began doing this work that I tapped into how all this maneuvering made me feel. It felt tight, exciting, stressful, and also very familiar. I would flow from one thing to the next like an artist walking the high wire who would then spring into the role of a circus aerialist. My shoulders felt constricted and up to my ears. However, the mere suggestion of creating a list or moving with a plan felt offensive. It felt as if those suggesting it attempted to rob me of home, or worse, my trusted statue clutched to my chest. Who am I? I am adaptable. Not because I want to be. But because I've had to be.

STATUES, A MEANS FOR SURVIVAL

The statue was my trauma response—anxiety—and, more important, a survival tool. You will hear me say this throughout our time together: Every living thing wants to survive, and so our brain and nervous system will find every possible way to do just that, survive. It will find ways to be the most intelligent person in the room, not because we necessarily want to be, but because if we are, we can protect ourselves from those who possess the potential to cause harm. And so we create survival tools and things to keep us safe (more on that later). Often, our tools for survival become so much a part of who we are that we become married to them, becoming one with our survival. We begin to resemble our survival mechanism, so much so that we can't even tell ourselves apart from them. So when we ask the question "Who am I?" we don't know or can't always fully place ourselves, because who we are has become so buried beneath the influence of the trauma, the need to keep safe after witnessing or experiencing harm, and all the things we have picked up along the way to survive. We don't fully know who we are because we haven't had a moment to see ourselves separate from what we've experienced and the tools we've adapted to survive the aftershocks. Who are you when you are not in survival mode?

I encourage you to take a fine-tooth comb through your obvious and not so obvious survival tools. Look not only at your "imperfections" but also at the parts by which you excel. Allow yourself to take notice of your subtle and everyday unintentional movements, the movements that feel most familiar and like home. Possibly even look at the specialties in which you take pride. In other words, take a comb to your superpowers. More than likely, they, too, are tied to your wound.

Maybe your survival tool kit is not being hypervigilant or one step ahead. Possibly it's closing yourself off to the world before it has the time or opportunity to do the same to you. Or maybe it's burying yourself in work or talent. Here's an example of this approach: Jane had emotionally unavailable parents, which made her susceptible to chasing approval, so now at work, she buries herself in her duties and capabilities to feel acceptance, validation, and the emotional stability she missed as a child.

Now, as we begin, is a great time to drop into yourself and ask what actions and patterns you have developed simply to survive. Recognize who you are—not what you do, but *who you are*—in this present moment. What state do you inhabit? Ego would often have you list vocation, but asking yourself this question and answering honestly may uncover more. That "more" is the start of who you are in this season, and that knowledge is critical to knowing yourself. What does your voice sound like when no one is around? What secrets does it whisper to you? How full or empty do you feel after hearing it?

Being able to distinguish between myself and the replica allowed me to show empathy and begin the journey of becoming my own place of refuge. I know what it feels like to look outside yourself for the safety that only we can give. Because safety begins with us, I can attest that everything else is null and void without cultivating this vital relationship. Without it, even when protection found its way into my life, I still didn't feel it, and it didn't matter because the repair and, most notably, the cultivation of becoming and growing my own safe space within me had yet to take shape. I had to become my first sanctuary, and I couldn't do so until I recognized my current state (i.e., getting to self-intimacy), a state heavily affected by my childhood self, and began the work from there.

Remember the statue? I held on to this sense of adaption until I tapped into how it made me feel. I want you, the reader, to ask yourself the same question. Examine the patterns that you naturally fall into. What personal trait do you possess that you take pride in but doesn't necessarily make you feel safe? When examining it, how does it make you feel? It wasn't until I tapped into this question that I noticed that the sensations I felt while springing into action and "adapting" felt eerily familiar to all the times I had to adjust and just go with it as a child. It felt familiar to the moments when I didn't have time to sit in stability or safety but instead had to move on to the next step quickly. I hated the feeling of being activated, but unknowingly continued to put myself in this space. Does this sound familiar? If so, know that the roots of your superpower no longer have to control how you currently practice it. For example, I now understand that being adaptable is a beautiful attribute *and* I do not have to live in a constant state of adaptation.

The same can be said regarding the professions we choose and the skill sets we lean toward. I became a doula because I love supporting people as they welcome new life into the world, *and* I naturally *love* protecting and keeping people safe. I began my journey of managing and safeguarding as a child. This particular skill set felt routine and natural. So, friends, I pose the same question I asked myself: Is it talent or survival? And more than likely, it can be both. Often our superpowers are birthed out of just that . . . survival. However, once you hear the answer, know that you are brave enough to dig until you hit bedrock. This foundation is where we begin to give ourselves the gifts that perhaps our younger self and current self need and deserve, an existence beyond our statues and imitations of safety. If you asked who I was, my answer would be "Hurt. I am hurt. I am afraid. Nice to meet you." To know me, I needed to know my wounds. Once I could see them, I could distinguish between how much of it was me and how much of it was the residue of early chaos.

Now I begin my day with intention. I write things down. I remind myself that I don't always have to adapt. And every time I move with purpose, I give my current self and younger self the emotional security, safety, and peace that I longed for so long ago. You can too. We all start somewhere. Perhaps here is your inception.

- Begin by shedding those fears of visiting the childhood wounds or black hole of your life.
- Next, take time to fully discover your origin of disruption or mother wound, the tear as a result of which things were never quite the same.
- Spend time with, understand, and hold your child self. This is the place where many of our disruptions and tears happen.
- Ask yourself the three questions: *Who am I? Where am I? How long have I been here?* Again, don't lean into what you *do*. Who *are* you?
- Notice the rituals, actions, and longing for control you've attached to as an adult. Name your statue. What is the survival tool that you have become one with? What is your first memory of resourcing this survival tool—your statue?

CHAPTER TWO

Living Sanctuary

I'll never forget one of my favorite births that I attended as a doula. This mama had labored for hours. She was now in her sixth hour. She would sway and move and moan beneath the dim lighting of the birth tub in her home. Her baby was close. We all knew it. She had arrived within her labor's transition, and she began to question her ability to birth her baby. She asked if she was "doing it right," if she was breathing correctly. Doubt had begun to sink in. The meditative song "Sanctuary" began to play. She and I both became lost in the trance of its lyrics.

The part that stood out for me was the last few lines: "I'll be a living sanctuary for you . . ." Seeing this mother, who had made it to nine months carrying her little one and now had arrived at a place of finally birthing the baby she had been carrying, allowed me to see the truth within the stanza. While we are living, breathing safe havens for one another, we must first be able to locate sanctuary within ourselves. This becomes easier to do once we've located and worked through our past wounds. I see developing a sense of self-sanctuary as the next step in self-intimacy. The more you are intimate with yourself and your past, the better you become at being sanctuary for yourself because you more clearly understand what you need.

What is a sanctuary? A sanctuary is a place of refuge or safety. Picture the safest space you have ever felt. Let's imagine it's a place. What does it smell like? Does it have walls and a ceiling, or is it limitless like the open sky? Does its texture feel like honey and magnolia, soft to the touch and sweet to the taste, its petals wrapping themselves around you gently? Maybe it's a color or a thought that brings ease. Perhaps it's a memory. Or a certain person's embrace. Maybe you have yet to experience an emotional or physical space that safety inhabited so fully or where it whispered the words "I know." And because of this, it isn't easy even envisioning a place so wonderful.

I want you to know that your sanctuary, your place of refuge and safety, is not some far-away dwelling attainable only to those whom the fates deem honorable. Sanctuary resides right here within us, doors cascading open as arms stretched wide, welcoming us home and drawing us near. It's so important to find sanctuary in ourselves after excavating those early wounds as it becomes our new point of reference. Instead of swiftly running back to our survivor tools, we can respond with a bit more intentionality and stillness to everyday situations that may trigger us when we've settled into authentic interior peace; when we've settled into sanctuary within.

IN SEARCH OF SANCTUARY

So how do we find this sacred temple in ourselves? First, we cease our labor of looking elsewhere and look inside. Many of our primary survival tools are demonstrated by grasping for quick fixes. Things feel tough; we look to our careers, children, and companions to stop the wound's bleeding and heal it. And while our external relationships can be a form of sanctuary, they are not and should not be our primary sanctuary, or what I'll call our first sanctuary. Why is it essential to form our sanctuary within? Because, unlike our external relationships, *we* are always with us. And that alone is a gift.

One may question, isn't self-intimacy—knowing ourself—the same as self-sanctuary? And to that, I offer that whereas self-intimacy is the process of unearthing the deep knowledge of ourself, self-sanctuary is the result, or its fruit. Sanctuary is what we discover has been there all along, in us as shelter, as we continue our self-intimacy practice.

Begin locating your sanctuary outside your moments of activation. My tool for locating sanctuary is in my breath. Often sanctuary is the opposite of your survival tools. For example, I found that when I am anxious, my survival tool is to become busier. My body feels fast and hot, and the only source of relief is to become more active and scattered. Remember, our survival tools often are our initial trigger go-to's. I've heard it said that urgency is a trauma response. So, if your answer (or survival tool) for fear or triggers is to become more urgent, try the opposite on for size. See what it feels like to sit quietly in the temporary chaos, knowing that it is temporary. While sitting in the fear and confusion, touch it while paying close attention to your breath. Slow down, slow your breathing down even though everything within your body wants to rush through.

DISMANTLE TO DISCOVER

If we want to thrive within our relationship with ourself and create a place of inner sanctuary, we must dismantle and disarm everything within our programming that prevents us from com-

ing into a surer sense of self. We must do away with the belief
that we should live in a perpetual state of longing. We are the
liberation that we long for. As adults, we tell ourselves we *know*
this, but it's rare that we continuously, intentionally *act* on this
knowing. I want you to change that. This is the space where self-
intimacy and self-sanctuary may seem to merge. While self-
intimacy is getting to know oneself deeply, self-sanctuary is then
creating a safe place for the authentic you to dwell both within
and outside yourself.

Often when we don't know ourself, all we can do is emote or
"treat" our symptoms of hurt and deprivation. We can't heal the
root if we haven't done the work or taken the deeper journey.
The more you take on self-intimacy as a practice, the more you
discover what you really need during life's great labors and that
you are the point person who can often provide yourself with the
necessary solace and relief. Right here. Right now.

While we began talking about self-intimacy in chapter 1, I'd
like to add to this framework. I believe there are three components of self-intimacy work: emotional, mental, and physical. All
are important and so very connected, and all lead to creating
sanctuary for oneself.

WHERE AM I? HOW LONG HAVE I BEEN HERE?

During my trip, I asked these questions: "Where am I?" and
"How long have I been here?" Knowing where we are and how
long we've been living within the emotional space is how we
begin on the path to cultivating emotional self-intimacy. Coming
out of my childhood experience, I felt like a soldier home from
war. Toys would fall, and my body would jump. I would become
easily startled by everyday loud noises. Much like me, my anxiety had also matured. When I finally began my own healing jour-

ney, I realized how long I had been dealing with the nonstop overthinking and what I call motor brain running on full steam. I'd flash back to being a small child, and the feeling of heaviness and darkness would set in. I'd feel as though I was in danger even when I was not and couldn't understand why. I remember walking up to the prayer lines at church wanting to be fixed—from what, I did not understand. Where was I? I was in a continual state of fear and apprehension. How long had I been here? Since I could remember.

The Buddhist nun Pema Chodron says, "Start where you are." For us to begin, we must know where we are. By answering these questions: "Who am I?" "Where am I?" "How long have I been here?" I was able to see where I was. I noticed that I needed support in breaking down and healing the trauma I'd experienced.

Emotional self-intimacy is understanding *why* we feel *what* we feel. Emotional self-intimacy asks where the need to avoid discomfort comes from. Truthfully, we want to get to the bottom of things quicker, but often we really just want the surfaced sensation to stop. I want you to know that getting to the bottom is just that. It means touching the root of it all, whispering the words "And there it is." Despite our greatest fears, it is exploring the chasm of where it all began.

Emotional self-intimacy digs for the true origin of our feelings. Example: You've spent numerous days and countless hours working on a project. And when presenting, you receive feedback that, although constructive, triggers feelings of rejection. A person with a matured emotional self-intimacy would be able to pinpoint that they weren't upset by the critical input but by the fact that what they worked so hard on wasn't accepted because they suffer from perfectionism and a fear of overarching rejection.

When we don't have the tools to explore what's hiding underground, we plant our origin flag upon the hill of the present, blaming what's happening now instead of the core cause. It's certainly more accessible. However, in the long run, it's not efficient or sustainable.

An example of someone who practices emotional self-intimacy would be:

1. They look for the root of their aboveground feelings. They accept that there may be more to the story beyond the initial thought, reaction, and emotion. They inquire inward first.
2. They understand that their feelings are theirs to own. And while they may have community and resources alongside them if and when needed, those who practice emotional self-intimacy understand that they gain so much more as they get to know themselves and own this exploration.
3. People who practice emotional self-intimacy can better advocate for themselves and communicate their needs. When you know what's at the center of your emotions, you can better share your genuine concern and actual needs instead of simply emoting. When I know why I feel what I feel, I can better communicate what I need and why.

How do we get there, to emotional self-intimacy? You will hear me say this a lot in this book, but it bears repeating. We allow ourselves to live in a constant state of curiosity and grace. We remain interested in the "why" of our feelings, emotions, reactions, and behaviors, and show ourselves immediate grace for them. This work will require that you know (really know in your bones) that you are unlocking the deep inner working of your why and what happened to you and in you, recently or so long ago. And to put it candidly, a lot of rich earth will surface. And when it does, know that sometimes our initial response and thoughts will likely resemble our survival tools and all that we are attempting to grow past. However, this is where the gift unfolds. After you've reeled and frayed, ask yourself, "Why?" And in this questioning, try not to focus on anything external outside yourself. This self-curiosity is where emotional self-intimacy is birthed.

YOUR NERVOUS SYSTEM AND SURVIVAL

When I began to do the work of emotional self-intimacy, asking myself the three questions that I asked in my trip, I realized the many ways that my nervous system was an equal shareholder in my relationship with self. Our nervous systems are biased and hellbent on not only protecting and keeping us safe but also getting our needs met. Our nervous system's MO is simply survival. Because of this, our nervous system puts in place responses to triggers, fears, and the past that we've experienced, all to keep us here, making sure that we survive. It remembers the broken places where damage has been done and reminds us fiercely that "it" happened. Again, our nervous system's goal is to protect and keep us safe. This protection may trigger panic, an unknown sense of threat or fear. If you experienced danger on the corner of Forty-fifth and Lincoln decades ago, it won't matter if where before was desolation and doom, now there is a newly erected theme park. Your nervous system will remember that danger lurked here in this place. Your nervous system, via triggers, may even advise you to avoid this now "happy place" altogether. Your nervous system reminds you that here in this place, harm happened, and there is still an ache to be tended.

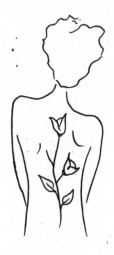

Roses and Garlic

I opened part 1 with a nod toward the relationship between roses and garlic for a reason. Gardening experts suggest planting these companion plants together. The garlic repels and protects the rose from pests like ants and aphids due to its strong smell. The garlic is also an antifungal, protecting the rose from all sorts of blights. This plant relationship is primarily one-sided, though. Rose doesn't do much for garlic. I like to refer to this plant couple as Rick and Gladys.

The 1980s "Super Freak" singer Rick James couldn't be more dissimilar from the soulful queen Gladys Knight. They are different in every way imaginable. While many enjoy taking in the smell of a bouquet of roses, the same is not necessarily true for garlic (unless it's in a pot of stew, of course). These two are opposites. However, garlic works hard and takes on the role of protecting rose. It wants to see her survive pestilence, fungal infections, and so much more.

Natural, and very human, emotions of disappointment, anger, sadness, or embarrassment can show up as garlic in our lives. The taste of anger repulses our society. However, anger can be the catalyst for change when allowed to express itself and not stuffed down and repressed. We try to fix sadness instead of allowing and welcoming it as the great teacher that it is, calling in and calling out what needs to be addressed. Sadness can be an opportunity for healing. The same is true for disappointment. Although pungent to taste, a lot like garlic, disappointment can be the very thing by which we are compelled to shift our energies, careers, and environment. When we don't allow the garlic of our lives to do its job, and we repress, press down, stuff, and fold away unpleasant sensations into deep closets, we risk being left unprotected. We attract the pestilence of self-sabotage, the blight of stagnation, and so much more.

In my own journey, it wasn't until I tasted the sadness and grief of having a miscarriage that I recognized the lack of support for those facing this sort of grief. It wasn't until I tasted the bitterness of disappointment over a childhood riddled with violence that I began to heal and mend my wounds. It wasn't until I tasted the fear of uncovering damage, shame, and blame and moved toward grace and forgiveness that I was able to see that we are all doing the best we can with the tools we have. When we allow the garlic in our lives to be aromatic, we can thrive just like the rose.

Regarding mental self-intimacy, our nervous systems provide the same care as garlic. You may ask, what's the difference between emotional and mental self-intimacy? I think of emotional self-intimacy as our garden's emotional root work. It is the door or entrance to our self-intimacy work. Most of us feel first and think second. In contrast, mental self-intimacy is the understanding and eventual mastery of our thoughts and their proper place. I like to categorize our thoughts into three types: hitchhiker thoughts, passenger thoughts, and driver's seat thoughts. Possessing mental self-awareness allows us to recognize and get in touch with all three.

#THOUGHTLIFE

I want you to know that a considerable part of becoming truly intimate with ourselves is becoming close with our thoughts, without judgment. We have been taught to stand in so much judgment of the inner voice within our heads. Our brain constantly offers feedback from what we perceive around us, as we take in both positive and negative messaging. The keyword here is "feedback," as it is not always fact. We pay attention and recognize the thoughts and treat them as passing traffic. Some thoughts are ours, and some are simply inherited from others and passing through. Once we have identified them, where do we want them to land? Recognizing the difference between the two clears the way for the thoughts we should give our attention to and those we can afford to let go and be on their way.

You've heard it said that the primary voice you hear throughout your day is the voice inside your head. Our thoughts are with us from the time we wake up until we are well into our dreams. Understanding how our thoughts and self-talk can keep us from connecting with our most authentic selves is vital. The first step is recognizing your thoughts and being able to call them by name: Hitchhiker, Passenger, or Driver's Seat. When we recognize where our thoughts categorically fall, we can better identify which thoughts to devote the proper energy toward and which ones we can wish well on their way.

Hitchhiker thoughts are just that. They are strangers, wandering along the open highway of our minds. You pick them up along the way, knowing that they are simply passing by with little to no emotional investment beyond getting from point A to point B. Once your hitchhiker is out of the car and on their way, that is the end of their journey. Examples of hitchhiker thoughts are the fleeting thoughts that jump into your mental vehicle from your current environment. Social media, that scary Lifetime movie about being abducted, or the person who cut you off in traffic. These are all things that may trigger hitchhiker thoughts. Though the slightest external stimuli can trigger hitchhiker thoughts, they are powerful.

Example: You are driving along when suddenly a fellow driver cuts you off in traffic. After the infraction, the driver proceeds to flip you off right as they put the pedal to the metal to add insult to injury. How do you feel? You feel offended and angry and are in utter shock by the stranger who has now left you, perhaps reeling in the dust. Your thoughts begin to run wild with what you would have said if that person were so brave as to find themselves face to face with you and how you would have let them know that they messed with the wrong person. You replay and replay and then reimagine some more. You picture yourself finding something noteworthy to say right as you leave *them* in the dust. Oh, how the tables have turned. You have now gotten the last word, and you are happy about it until you remember that this is not how everything went down, and the hitchhiker thought that perhaps enters is, once again, "You don't matter." *Everyone always* does _____ to you. You need to be more like _____. Because this would *never* happen to _____.

When you finally arrive at your destination, you feel heavy and exhausted from all the hypothetical conversations you would have had with the stranger. The mental tension is palpable, and currently, your day is influenced. This domino effect is the power of the unseen and unrealized hitchhiker thought. When unaware of these thoughts and their potential emotional impact on our day, we further dive into the rabbit hole of these feelings and entertain the thoughts more than they deserve. Suppose we can simply see and recognize these thoughts as minor interruptions triggered by the temporary of our environment. By calling these thoughts by name and labeling them as merely hitchhikers passing through, we can shift our energies to the ideas that really matter within our cognitive space, to the thoughts that are worthy of investigation rather than a swift drop-off.

Then there are passenger thoughts. Imagine going on a road trip with a friend. The intent of the road trip is for you to go to the same terminus. Perhaps when you reach your destination, you stay together, or maybe your passenger is just a ride-along. Sometimes our passengers are people we invited. Other times, they may have invited themselves. I remember taking many road trips home from college with roommates, friends, or that classmate who you sort of knew that lived close to your hometown. We've all been there when on the road you immediately regret agreeing to the rideshare arrangement and can't wait for your passenger's exit to arrive. Passenger thoughts are those that were perhaps influenced by your upbringing, childhood, and overall lived experience. They can sometimes keep you on course, sometimes weigh you down.

Your life's experience, environment, societal voice, and those around you form many of your passenger thoughts, such as right versus wrong, shaping how you now perceive the world. Perhaps it was implied growing up that you had to get married, because how else would you be complete? You have to have children because that's what women do. Maybe society whispered in your ear that your body is not a beautiful one. Or your hair is not good hair. Or that you are unholy because of who you love. Our passenger thoughts permeate us and are often introduced to us in subtle yet impactful ways. Like the passenger who carpools, passenger thoughts can be invited or uninvited. They impact our point of view and, occasionally, the lens through which we see reality. Passenger thoughts ride with us, going in the same direction until we arrive at the road's end. Our mental self-intimacy work looks like a dialogue with our thoughts. It asks their name and where they are journeying from. Remember we talked about naming our wounds? We do this by asking for our thoughts' names and listening to what they say.

Example: You may have difficulty stepping away from work, whether for leisure or simply because it's time to stop. You judge yourself harshly when you need to tend to your basic needs while working, and you consistently feel that you need to do more. The passenger thought that enters is "You are not working hard enough." You can't possibly step away. A practice of mental self-awareness would be asking the passenger thought, "What's your name? Where are you coming from?" If we give ourselves a moment to sit still and listen, the cool thing is that our thoughts will answer. In this case, it may say, "My name is second grade failed science project." You can then respond in kind, "I am no longer in second grade, nor is this a science project," letting the passenger thought out of your car.

We can inquire (curiosity is key) of our passenger thoughts at any point. Ask, "Does this way of thinking still serve who I am today? Do I still believe this way of thinking to be true?" When you receive your answer, know that you can part ways. You do not have to continue to ride alongside an unwanted (perhaps newly realized uninvited) passenger.

You occupy the driver's seat. As drivers, we decide who we allow in and what thoughts can continue along the journey. We choose the beliefs to which we offer our energy. When we recognize that the rumination of what we would have said to the lady who cut us off in traffic is a hitchhiker thought simply looking for a place to land—that this feeling and brief interruption in our day is temporary, and it would prove futile to invest our mind in someone who more than likely has moved on with their day—we can then release the hitchhiker thought on its way and refocus our energy on ourselves, not allowing what just happened to take hold of us or how we view ourselves the rest of our day.

When you have spent a considerable amount of time on social media playing the comparison game, and now you're not feeling successful enough, you hear the hitchhiker thoughts whispering,

"You are not worthy enough, lovable enough, flourishing or producing enough." When we know that this is just a hitchhiker thought looking for a ride, and that it is not ours nor truth but simply triggered from our most recent environment and messaging, we can let it pass along without claiming it as ours to keep.

When we recognize the origin and pressure to work more and be more, forsaking rest, as passenger thoughts that found their way to us from our upbringing and societal influences, we can then recognize that those thoughts are not the truth and view them as ideas that perhaps we didn't even ask for and were pushed upon us. We can thank the passenger thoughts for the parts that helped us achieve, *and* we can pull over and let them out at the nearest exit when we witness how some of those thoughts no longer align with our core beliefs and who we are today.

This idea, in practice, can be a visualization exercise:

1. Stop the car. Similar to how you wouldn't let a passenger out of a moving vehicle, the same is valid when releasing the ways of thinking that no longer serve us. Stopping (or pausing) will also purposefully disrupt the path that you are currently traveling.

2. While stopped, recognize and acknowledge the space the passenger thought occupied and your attachment to it. Recognize how much room you will have within the soon-to-be-vacant seat to do with what you will. Ask yourself, "What would I like to replace this thought with? What thoughts feel more in unison with who I am today?" Or you may want to leave the seat empty until you find what feels more authentic to your current personal beliefs.

3. Open the door so you can release the maladaptive passenger thought *and* welcome more aligned thoughts.

Again, we are the driver. We determine who continues to ride along in the car of our mind. Remember, when we are distracted by our passenger or hitchhiker thoughts, we also become inattentive to our actual destination or true path.

Understanding the role of our nervous system and how it sustains us is vital. Similar to garlic, our nervous system affects our thought patterns even as it is there to protect and act as a companion helping our survival. It is there to ensure that our needs are met and that we prevail. I like to think of our nervous system as the class secretary of our body, consistently taking notes and cues from our past and ensuring we stay safe. Unfortunately, I heard a therapist say that we don't know how our nervous system will show up for us. And this is why the work is so important. When we are aware of ourselves (who we are, where we are, how long we have been in this space), we can characterize the garlic in our lives, recognize its potential not only to protect us but to grow us.

The approach to this work will look different for everyone, calling for a bottomless plunge into your journey and examining your wounds, implementing various modalities that we will explore together. As mentioned, this quest may take many shapes and forms. Your path toward healing may shapeshift and bend. In my experience, I found that one path and discovery would often wind toward and into another. Almost as if all passageways were conspiring to make me whole.

Wherever you begin, know that this journey is a continued work. There is the care and checking in and pruning back and flourishing. It is a transformation from reactiveness into a daily ritual, a prompt and reminder to keep your feet planted here in the present. When we are in the present, we can approach our past as the person we are now, tending to the roots with our current tools.

I hope that you fall.
A fall that lands you deeply within yourself.
Knowing yourself
So that you can distinguish between the garlic that is present
    to guide . . .
and the weeds growing wild.

PHYSICAL SELF-INTIMACY

Our self-intimacy work applies to the physical element as well. I define physical self-intimacy as the awareness of one's body, its safety, and its right to autonomy in this world. It is the space felt to explore yourself without shame or judgment. It is how comfortable or at home we feel within our bodies. The safety and ownership we feel in our bodies is vital for our thriving.

Eventually, my mother would leave my father when I was ten years old and marry my stepfather, Ronald, a brown-skinned man with bold features and an infectious laugh. He was funny with a bright smile, loud and boisterous. I liked him, and my mother instantly fell head over heels in love with him. They married six months after meeting. And just like that, my life and my mother's and sister's lives drastically changed.

I went from having only one sibling to three additional stepsiblings, two stepsisters and a stepbrother. I went from hearing fights and my father's abuse in the middle of the night to all of the violence dissipating as if it were never there to begin with. My stepfather was a religious man involved in the church, and so had become my mother. Our lives became filled with Sunday morning and midweek services. Whenever the doors were open, I was at the church house where I'd hear sermons about our bodies not being our own but being bought with a price. We were told that we all must deny the flesh and that it was abhorrently evil on its own. As an adolescent, I gathered that this flesh of mine was bad and worthy of being ignored and forsaken. I internalized that actions birthed from the flesh in and of itself were bad, as were my thoughts. You too?

This messaging perpetuated, I think, many people's lack of physical self-intimacy within the environment. How was I supposed to get to know my physical self when this body of mine was something in which I was repeatedly told I had no ownership? How could I become intimate with something while also being asked to forsake and abandon it? How do I become one with this body, knowing it fully, while cursing its flesh? It is impossible to become intimate with anything that you do not know. And it is even harder to know something you do not own.

Many passenger thoughts were gathered from my early years in church that I would later have to open the door for to let out of the car. The church's teachings influenced how I thought and felt about my body. And while all of this is an unfortunate truth, the marriage between my mother and stepfather, Ronald, had its upsides, as it gifted me an experience that I had yet to have in the early parts of my childhood, a peaceful home. My mother and Ronald had married in a small wedding after church. They were both overjoyed to start their new life together. Truthfully, I was excited too. I'd relocated from small-town Sylacauga to what the small-town folks called the big city, Birmingham, and had finished my second year of middle school. It was the summer before my eighth-grade year. I was a small kid and had just about hit puberty, but not quite.

I was happy about my parents' marriage. Until this point, I

had only seen relationships mired with trauma and violence, adults who didn't know how to disagree without resorting to putting their hands on each other. My mother's side of the family was the functional one. They had regular homes where children went to bed without overhearing cries for relief from pain and misery. There I could be a kid, not activated and on constant alert to protect those around me. I could be free.

After my mother's marriage to my stepfather, peace seemed to be my new normal. Things were good. I was introduced to new extended family members and they welcomed me with open arms. They all seemed friendly. They laughed loudly, cracking jokes at each other. Around this time, I was introduced to one of my stepfather's uncles, Ned. He was an older man with gray hair and seemed kind. He was one of the few people who took in my stepfather, Ronald, when he was homeless. He was a bit of a recluse and stayed at home more often than not. When my parents were between apartments, we would spend the night there. One morning I found his secret stash of 1960s *Playboy* magazines hidden between his more acceptable magazines.

After my parents found our tiny apartment, we'd visit him after church just to say hello. I remember Uncle Ned frying us up a bologna sandwich for lunch during one such visit. I watched as he pressed the mystery meat to the pan, instructing me that the way you know that bologna is finished cooking is by the bubbles that would reveal themselves along the edges. He had the demeanor of a grandparent, and I think I hoped in my heart for an adult figure of that nature who was safe and trustworthy.

One evening, my parents decided to have a night out. By this time, they had become heavily involved in the church. This evening, some preacher was speaking at a revival. Arrangements were made for my sister and me to stay with Uncle Ned. They dropped us off and said their goodbyes as we put our overnight bags down by Ned's floral sofa. We had already eaten dinner and came in our pajamas, ready to watch a movie and then go to bed. Ned made a pallet on the floor for my sister and me. My sister and I lay on the floor watching television and chatting between ourselves as he sat in his living room chair, looking on until we both fell asleep.

When I awoke, I felt a body next to me that was not my sister's. I felt the hands of an adult touch me, but not a touch that I had experienced from the adults in my life. This touch wasn't a slap or the loving touch of the new adults I had recently met. This touch felt like heartache and loss of the little bit of trust I had left for adults and those around me. I felt a hand go under my pajamas. I froze. I didn't know what to do. My eleven-year-old mind started racing a million miles a minute. Time arrested itself in its tracks. I had heard stories and my fair share of after-school specials on "bad touch." However, somehow, I was now in the after-school movie. I imagined little Peggy, Jack, and Jill, from the movies; they had all made their way to the "bad stranger's" van, house, or sketchy alley after school on the sitcoms. All of these shows seemed predictable, building to an assault of some sort about to take place. However, for this I was not prepared. I wasn't in a stranger's van or the far side of town playing hooky. These sitcoms often painted the victim as unknowingly yet obviously walking into the hands of danger and its predatory clutches. I was here, in my "new uncle's" living room, now a victim of molestation and the complete loss of trust in everyone.

I jumped up, ran to the bathroom, and locked the door. I froze again. Where do I go from here? Was this my fault? Why would a grown-up do this? Is he going to hurt me? What happens now? I couldn't leave, and I felt trapped in both the fear of what would happen next and the walls surrounding me. I looked for a window to escape the predator in the other room. Could I walk for help? Where would I go? He seemed so kind before.

Suddenly I remembered that my younger sister was still in the living room. I had to go back in there. She was only five years old. I couldn't be sure that he wouldn't try to do the same thing to her.

I unlocked the door and proceeded to walk back to the living room. Ned was now sitting in his bedroom, enveloped by the dark. The pitch black around him was as if what was inside of him decided to sit beside him instead. I saw his shadow move as he asked me to come and sit with him. He apologized and then proceeded to hug me, pulling my eleven-year-old body onto the bed with him. I managed to push him away and walk out of the bedroom. He followed me to the living room. I remember not being sure what was most disturbing—the fact that he had molested me or that he was so calm, maintaining his voice below a whisper. I was sure that he'd done this before, and that I was just a number in the long list of traumas unleashed by his pedophilic hands. Ned asked me not to tell and apologized again. I promised not to speak of it.

Once he left the room, I lay back down on my pallet, pretending to fall asleep. I had a plan, and that was to escape. I waited. Luckily the old-school tan-colored rotary phone was next to our pallets on the coffee table. Minutes later, I reached for the phone to call my parents. I hoped they would answer. It was late and past midnight. I didn't know what to do, necessarily. But I knew that I couldn't spend the night there in that house. I prayed, "Please pick up the phone." "Hello?" I whispered into the phone. "Come get me now." My parents replied, "Is everything okay?" I can still hear the developing panic in their voices. All that I could manage to say was, "Come get me." I quickly and quietly hung up and returned to my pallet, next to my sister, who was still asleep and unaware of what had taken place. Ten minutes later, and in what felt like an eternity, I saw the headlights of my parents' car shining through the window and made a run for the door, leaving my pallet and overnight bag behind.

For you to heal it
You have to feel it.

I carried the trauma of being molested for years afterward. I ran out of the house and into my family's car. My stepfather, Ronald, went into the house to gather my sister and talk to the new uncle. My mother asked me questions like "What happened? Did he touch you? Are you okay?" My words sat stuck at the base of my throat, refusing to make their way out of my mouth. What happened? I didn't know. Did he touch me? Words failed to escape my mouth as I attempted to answer yes. "Are you okay?" Was I? How could I be? Are we ever okay after something like this happens? This short and frantic conversation would be the last of the talks concerning what happened to me that night.

I had barely trusted the adults to keep me safe before this, and after experiencing this trauma, it was hard for me to trust anyone. I was violated. Sexually assaulted. I still remember the predatory way he waited for me to fall asleep, similar to how an animal waits for its prey, except in this case lurking in plain sight, waiting for its victims to be most vulnerable, or in my case, asleep as a child. After the molestation, there was this strange silence. My parents didn't talk about it ever again. At least not to me. And what the adults don't talk about, kids often absorb as a secret to be kept, locking it away and tossing the key.

After this, I stopped hugging adults. I was too afraid to show affection or my childlike admiration toward all who encountered me. It would take years for me to be okay with any attachment, touch, or pat on the back. Even hugs from those that meant well could trigger the memory of that evening. Being a victim of molestation changed me. It changed the way I perceived the world as a child. It changed the relationship I had with my body. Everyone was now a stranger. Ronald would ask me if I was okay, and nothing more. My parents did nothing, they neither spoke of the molestation nor pressed charges, and that newly acquired relative proceeded with his life as if nothing had happened.

I would still have to see Ned from time to time. One time he came over to our home with a friend and I was quickly hurried to the front door by my mother, as if I wouldn't see him sitting in our living room, on our furniture. I'm not sure what he was doing at our home. I know how it made me feel. After what he did to me, his presence in my home made me feel worthless. My parents not doing anything about the monster who touched their daughter, but allowing him into their home, echoed, "Brandi, you don't matter. Your emotional and physical safety don't matter. Your feelings don't matter." I now think of what it would've meant to me if my parents had done something about it, or even talked more about it, thus freeing me from keeping an unspoken secret.

As a kid, I pondered what was worse, the molestation or the fact that my parents did nothing. I'm still not sure.

The small and few places that seemed to be safe were no longer. I felt displaced within my body, my first home. This is what trauma does. It separates us from ourselves, leaving us without a home. And I wrestled and foraged in search of it. Maybe you did not experience sexual assault but your body has been made to feel like something you didn't have full autonomy over in other ways.

On the way to practicing physical self-intimacy? Ask yourself: How do I process somatic feelings (those regulated to the body as opposed to the mind) and sensations? Do I hold them, cast them away in judgment, or do I experience a shutdown prohibiting me from exploring deeper? Do I feel numb?

Although cultivating physical self-intimacy may initially begin with dissecting, disassembling, and deconstructing our passenger thoughts about our bodies, the ongoing work is also practiced daily. This kind of intimacy is how we see and sometimes, for the first time, become acquainted with ourselves from *our* perspective instead of from the perspective and beliefs of others. The practice of physical self-intimacy arises every time we are told we should be taller or more petite, different from what we are. Physical self-intimacy arises when we move from shame around our body's sexuality and desires to a place of love and acceptance. Physical self-intimacy is the ability to dispel the myths we were told about our bodies, reclaiming our bodies as our own. In practice, other people's opinions of my body and how it presents out in the world have nothing to do with me and no longer pull rank in how I view myself. How you see my body and how I see my body, the two no longer carry the same weight.

Physical intimacy requires us to rend asunder the words that made this flesh feel less than adequate, and our bodies feel less than holy, seen, and celebrated. Take notice of how your body responds to this freedom, of the sensations felt as you release one by one the tales told and unhealed wounds projected toward your body.

Finish this sentence: In my body I feel _____.

Maybe for you the answer is "In my body I feel exhausted." What is causing the exhaustion? And what might you do to counter it? What can you do to create sanctuary for your physical self when bodily you are feeling the effects of stress, worry, or doubt? We must cultivate self-intimacy *first,* for many reasons and many personal benefits.

Reason #1 is easy as Sunday morning and so very true: When we grow self-intimacy in all forms, we have an acute awareness of what we want and what is essential. When we know these two things, even when conflicted, we can always come back to ourselves and know what we need to nurture ourselves and to thrive.

Reason #2: When we have a sense of self-intimacy, we are aware of our limits and capabilities. When we know these things, there's a bit less scurrying after things that perhaps matter and make everyone else happy but leave you depleted and worn. The same is true for our capabilities. When we know our faculty, we can differentiate from the inner voice that may be negative environmental feedback and become our own hype man.

Reason #3: When we connect with ourselves in such an intimate way, when interacting with those around us, we can prioritize our sense of equity in shared spaces, knowing how much of something is ours and how much of the load is someone else's baggage to carry.

We *are* our first and most valuable love. Cultivating self-intimacy in all forms (emotional, mental, and physical) is part of a captivating process that leads you to self-sanctuary. Why? Because when we are in an intentional state of discovery, asking ourselves the hard questions that may not emerge from the rubble on their own, we open ourselves up in a way that many seldom do. We begin to live in the present, truly experiencing this life. I see so many people where life is happening around them and to them. In this fast-paced world that we live in, we can all fall into this pattern of reaction and projections, of emoting without stopping to ask ourselves "What's really going on here?" However, it is super important that when life gets to lifing, this is the moment when we must remember our place in the driver's seat, checking in with all of the sectioned-off territories of ourselves, the apparent parts and the pieces that were long forgotten, being curious about what's happening in us in that very moment.

This deep-rooted practice of not simply being what I call "lifed" all over the place but being curious about how life is showing up within us and how our bodies are feeling around it, how it resurfaces things within our mental space, and in our emotions, is how to begin laying the foundation for self-sanctuary. Because when we can pinpoint what's happening inside and outside us and differentiate between ourselves and the triggered chaos, we can act as a safe harbor, a sanctuary for ourselves, gifting ourselves with everything we need at that moment to continue in a way that will grow us forward. When we discover the roots, we can tend to the leaves and everything on the surface more efficiently.

For me, self-sanctuary looks like getting out in nature and touching it. It looks like grounding myself in meditation and breathing. When life feels overwhelming and complicated, I focus on the question "What do I really want? What is my most uncomplicated and most attainable heart's desire?" Usually, the answer that my spirit whispers back is simple. You know, the basics—food, water, shelter, and to do the things I love. And that answer refocuses me in a moment of chaos.

What does your spirit whisper back to you? Within that whisper is where self-sanctuary is found.

1. What has acted as the garlic in your life? How has your nervous system reacted to try to keep you safe and what might you want to change about this reaction?
2. Identify an area of self-intimacy where further work may be needed. Is it in your emotional, mental, or physical intimacy?
3. What does inner sanctuary feel like for you? Now give that feeling more attributes with the five senses. What do you see, smell, feel, taste, hear in your personal sanctuary?

CHAPTER THREE

Partnership as a Great Teacher

P latonic and romantic relationships serve as great teachers in our lives. I've found that our relationships not only teach us about those we are in relationship with, but they also reveal profound and undiscovered mysteries about ourselves. They are a direct mirror, reflecting the areas we might otherwise not see, introducing us to a crash course in further self-awareness. During the most challenging moments in my relationships, I've questioned if I was meant for such a task as being in relationship. Been there? There were just too many uncontrollable variables and unknown outcomes to calculate. When you've experienced deep wounds, even when you are aware of them and know how to locate your inner sanctuary, allowing people into the innermost sanctum of your life can still be hard. Being in relationship teaches us that there are more things outside of our control than within it. To love is to also willfully and, hopefully, wisely surrender to this truth.

Relationships reveal the areas where we've felt unworthy of love, care, and being fully seen. I'm sure you've witnessed it before. The one friend who is there for everyone else. Who tends to everyone else's injuries except their own. This may be the role they've had to occupy since time's inception. But what happens when *their* well feels depleted? This is where self-intimacy, sanctuary, and our external relationships meet. This is where our relationships can teach us that to love ourselves, we must allow others to care for us as well. Our relationships reveal the places we've known to be strong and no longer have to be. The areas hardened with calluses from old wounds that our relationships show still need mending, still need softening. Much like life's instructor, our relationships are not all blissful feelings but also hard lessons learned, bringing out our inner child and the areas that have not been heard or healed.

Healthy relationships teach us that we are worthy of protection and that our needs are not a burden but a call for love. I saw this teacher in the kitchens of my grandmother Juril and my aunties. When my mother needed protection from my father's abuse, she could find shelter among her cousins and aunties. This taught me the power of the relationships we possess in sisterhood gatherings, kitchen covens, and front porches filled with real and play cousins; these relationships hold us in comfort and act as co-laborers in our thriving, joy, and healing. And while these relationships are not bound together by a piece of paper and I-do's, there is no lack of commitment and devotion present. There is an unspoken yet demonstrated agreement of unconditional love and support, whether through meals prepared when loved ones are sick or experiencing hard times. These relationships are tried and true.

We make promises to be there, to have and to hold, to love and cherish. I learned through these connections that to be in a relationship is a daily choice and a commitment to be honored. And that our platonic relationships are just as sacred. The connections I witnessed amongst the women in my family taught me to cultivate and value these relationships as much as any other. As a little girl, they showed me the deepest kind of enchantment and healing that any relationship can wield. They taught me how to nurture well, and that attachment and nurturing are needs as basic as food and water.

One of the crucial things I've learned through relationships is that to be in relationship is to not only know and learn love for others but to ultimately learn how to love ourself. Being in relationship has taught me that even when surrounded by an abundance of love, no one can love me the way I love me, and to search for such love outside myself is futile. I had yet to fully learn and appreciate this lesson before meeting my husband, Jon.

Jon and I married young. We were mere teenagers, only eighteen and nineteen, when we met. We fell hard, fast, and like a body of water, so very effortlessly. Our love was easy, it felt like a Sunday kind of love. Immediately, Jon's arms felt like home. My heart was his. Despite this deep connection, it would be well into our partnership before he and I would begin cultivating the intimacy we assumed had been present way back when. How could we be intimate with each other when our self-intimacy had yet to be birthed individually? The short answer: There wasn't a chance in hell. My marriage is the first place I learned to heal.

When Jon and I met, it was like a calm stream of knowing that I had found my person. He was gentle, subtle, and the stillness that I had longed for as a child. We met at Belmont University in the autumn of 2001. He and I would spend late nights listening to Stevie Wonder, dissecting every lyric. Questioning what the songwriter meant when he wrote "Summer Soft." What did he mean when he referenced the season of winter rain? Jon would try his hand at explaining. I would listen, soaking in the fact that I had found a friend who loved the music of Stevie as much as I, to the point of studying every single word.

We'd go on to marry in a Nashville church gym just four years after first meeting. I was twenty-three and he twenty-two years old when we formed our union. (Upon reflection, this was probably too damn young.) Our wedding was filled with those we had acquired along the way of our early-twenties friendships. A friend sewed my dress. Jon rented his suit from the local tuxedo shop. After exchanging our vows, I remember thinking, "Well, that was easy. Perhaps too easy?" And so began our partnership. True story, we honeymooned in the exotic isles of Atlanta. We used whatever money we pooled from our wedding gifts to pay for our stay in Georgia. We were young and broke. But we had love, and for us, that was enough.

Our wedding night was a hot mess. Because of our upbringing, religious culture, and, for me, the need to "do it right" (i.e., wait until marriage), we were both inexperienced virgins. The sex talk for Jon involved "Don't you bring no babies home," and for me, "Save yourself because that's what you are supposed to do." And so I did. I'd had my handful of friends from school who became mothers well before entering their junior year of high school. I still remember the stares reverberating from the adults in judgment as my friends would walk by, bellies big and round. I didn't know if it was the penetrating looks from the teachers shaking their heads in disbelief or the way that my friends became a cautionary tale overnight. Due to this fear, there I was on my wedding night, scouring for which hole was the right hole. I was so unacquainted and unfamiliar with my body and its own pleasure. Because "good girls" didn't touch themselves, let alone have sex. Pleasure was reserved for the activation of our husbands. Jon and I fumbled for days attempting to figure out our bodies' jigsaw.

Our marriage began before we had time to catch up. At the time, we lived in a small apartment in Nashville, on Twenty-first Avenue. At best, our place couldn't have been more than 600 or 700 square feet. Our furnishings consisted of our bed, some records on the wall, and Jon's leopard futon, which he had purchased for his very first apartment post-college. The vinyl records were stuck to each other and to the wall by sticky glue and grit, much like our introduction to married life. Our home was small, but ours nonetheless.

I would become pregnant just three months after saying "I do." Jon and I met this shift from just the two of us to the three with joy and fear, as we had yet to enjoy our time as newlyweds. The prep work, especially the inner work, I had needed to do before becoming a partner, let alone before becoming a mother, was not in place. We did our best. We explored how to love each other while enmeshed in the vines of our early-twenties jungle. Like most of our age, we were winging adulthood. The entangled mess between discovering ourselves individually and each other as partners didn't help. Learning to love ourselves with our unhealed childhood wounds was the most challenging part and would eventually forage its way within our partnership. I would look to Jon for my need for safety, and Jon would search for his need for connection within me. From the beginning of our marriage, our deficits danced with each other as we searched for our childhood needs to be met. We were both looking for a balm of protection to wash over our childhood wounds.

TURTLING AS PROTECTION

Before entering my path of self-healing work, I would find myself often triggered in my romantic and platonic relationships; as one does when trauma is left unresolved. The seven-year-old girl, still afraid and still hiding under the table during her parents' fights, would emerge during moments of conflict, searching for safety. I would begin my hunt for the adults in the room, and there Jon was. He seemed safe and level-headed, characteristics that I was actively searching for and had rarely experienced. During most conflicts, I would stuff down my emotions and turtle, similar to a young child who had yet to find her voice. Keeping the peace was my goal as I performed this emotional disappearing act. Imagine what turtles do when they find themselves in danger. They go within their shell, coming out only when the coast is clear and the threat of danger is gone. This turtling, for me, looked like self-isolation, which I needed to quiet the discomfort. Why would I turtle? Although physical violence was no longer a part of my reality, I proceeded with life as if a fight or violence could break out at any moment, simply from my expression of disagreement, communicated hurt, or transparent feelings. If a conversation was too uncomfortable, I would turtle, bury my feelings within my shell, and proceed on to the next. Perhaps you can relate? My reason for turtling was protection. And it's not just protection from violence but from the threat of being unloved, unaccepted, or vulnerable. During moments of disagreement, I would retire into my hard shell and offer no words or thoughts. I would remove myself from the conversation, if not physically, I'd simply shut down. If you didn't know what I was thinking or feeling, you couldn't weaponize my feelings and vulnerability. Sound familiar? Turtling can look like:

- Emotionally shutting down. Using words that indicate indifference when indifference is not the case. Example: "I don't care," "It doesn't matter," when one's body language says otherwise.
- A semblance of physical and emotional self-isolation to avoid conflict and/or vulnerability.
- Our nervous system's flight response (emotional avoidance and/or physical disappearing) and freeze response (feeling frozen in place, where you can't move and the words simply won't come out).

I would retire into my shell, filled with inner dialogue and the complicated conversations I wished to be bold enough to have. These conversations would stay within the shell, afraid to call the words forward. To open my mouth would be to open myself up to possible hurt or disappointment, both of which I felt too fearful of experiencing any more than I already had. I have since learned that if, as a child, you were forced to navigate your emotions on your own or weren't provided emotional safety to process your feelings in the company of others, chances are, as an adult, you more than likely continue on with this behavior. Now, you may find yourself stifling your words and feelings, hiding them away, even when in a safe environment, even when welcome, and even as an adult. This retreating behavior, in turn, looks like the turtling described, self-isolating, hiding while you "figure it out," or even the offensive nature referred to as the silent treatment or ghosting. When triggered, I would look for Jon to be the safe space my early childhood lacked. Only he could call me from my shell.

Our relationship swayed from good to survival mode so very often within our first decade. It took until year fourteen to come to some understanding on how to love each other and raise a family, but since we'd wed so young we were both trying to grow up alongside a marriage. We were young, gifted, Black, and at times broke, attempting to raise our baby while pursuing our passions. I genuinely loved us and how we could dream. Collectively, we were fearless. We were each other's collaborators and partners. And we were just stubborn enough that for us, nothing was impossible.

Jon was a musician, so he traveled as I cared for our son, Jax. Jon would have some well-paying gigs, some not so much. He would produce music projects and tour to help supplement our income. I worked at a quaint shop in Nashville. We did whatever it took to "be the adults." Our identities as adults had yet to be discovered, and here we were, managing how to put food on the table.

Four years into our marriage, we would pack our belongings for a cross-country move to Los Angeles. We both decided it was time for us to try something new. We wanted to see if L.A. would be as kind to us as Nashville and if it would propel us further in our dream careers. So we packed all of our belongings into a shared 22-foot truck with friends who were also moving to L.A. Into the car we plopped, just the two of us with our then two-year-old, Jaxon. We wanted to create a better life for him. A life where he saw his parents go after their pursuits for him.

The grass was not initially greener on the other side of the country. We traveled for four days straight before reaching Los Angeles with $750 in our bank accounts and a profound un-awareness of a pending economic recession. We moved into a matchbox apartment in Los Feliz. And because Jon had picked up a job as bank teller in Nashville after getting screwed by an artist on payment, he could simply transfer from one branch to the other upon our arrival in Los Angeles. Jon took the train to work, and I used what we referred to as our Ford "Exploder," it was far beyond its mileage and in desperate need of repair, but it was all we had. Our then toddler had no clue about his parents' bet on themselves to win and succeed. To swim, not sink.

CHILDHOOD WOUNDS IN RELATIONSHIP

The first few years of our marriage were so rooted in our survival we had no time to dig and really decide how we wanted to raise ourselves or this family we were establishing. And even when we were finding ourselves financially beyond survival, we were still emotionally battling the wounds of our childhood.

I saw the battle in fragmented pieces with Jon. He appeared to want to be something or someone I didn't know. It was as if my presence was somehow crashing against the person he now wanted to be, which was single, not yet a father. He seemed to be craving all the parts of his early twenties he didn't get a chance to explore. The more he leaned into this unrecognizable figure, the less of a safe space he became. And truthfully, this fragmentation was only sometimes apparent. From my point of view, our days were mostly normal, with one version of Jon, and then there were moments where I would feel duplicity peeking through the fog.

Once this began, within the same four years, I started to have dreams and visions that warned me things were awry in our relationship. I would wake up in a cold sweat in the middle of the night and share with Jon how cruel he was in my dreams. In response, he dismissed them as mere fiction. However, like a trusted confidante, my dreams were warning, preparing, and divulging Jon's secrets. My intuition chose to tell me everything that I needed to know but wasn't ready to hear. And while I'm not sure what made me ready one Saturday morning for the answer, something had shifted. I wanted the truth. And more specifically, I wasn't afraid. I welcomed truth, flaws and all.

It was a typical Saturday morning. I had just finished visiting with a birth client and was returning home. Jon picked me up after having taken our now two younger boys to the park. By this time, they had both fallen asleep in the backseat. We began with our "Hey, loves" and "How are yous" as we started our ride together. We shuffled through the remaining events and schedule of the day, remembering that we had to do one more thing. As Jon drives, I use his phone, scrambling to find the event's details. I find them. However, I notice Jon's body as I rummage through his cellphone, innocently searching for the elusive email we both hoped to locate. He seemed anxious and uncomfortable. But why? He reaches for the phone and quickly closes it out, blackening its screen as I notice an email flash across his phone from an unknown sender.

I ask, "Who is this?"

He replies, "Who?"

I ask to see the phone.

He feels reluctant.

And although in this moment, Jon couldn't have felt less recognizable, I still knew him. I was familiar with the lines of his face and the furrow of his brow. I was familiar with how his eyes raised when he felt uncomfortable, and with the positioning of his body when he was afraid. He offered me his phone, and I began to scroll through text message after text message and email after email, and soon discovered what my dreams had whispered. Jon felt duplicitous because he was. He'd cheated and had been cheating for years. How could I have not known? As my fingers scrolled, what I knew as my life changed instantaneously. Should I leave? Should he leave? I didn't know what my next step would be. Unfortunately, there isn't a manual for heartbreak or betrayal of trust. After over a decade of marriage, we had gone from friends to lovers to now strangers.

Some people know what they will do when a transgression of this magnitude is committed. And while I would like to say that the revelation of Jon's infidelity and duplicity was sudden, the bottomless knowing was not.

Truth as Garlic

Truth comes in many forms. For me, it came by way of a text message. For you, it may come from a long past due exchange. However it comes, truth is also like the garlic mentioned in the previous chapter. Truth, although bitter at times, is here for your growth and highest good.

I'm not sure what made me more or less ready for the truth at that point in my relationship. I could have ignored the gut feeling to ask about the message that appeared across Jon's screen, but I chose not to and to follow my intuition. Back then, I had not yet started any intentional self-actualizing work. Perhaps my questioning and not accepting answers thrown to me like scraps called fearlessness forward. Somewhere between the questions and tug-of-war between truth and the debris of Jon's words, I knew that I would be okay, no matter how reality presented itself.

I emotionally battered myself black and blue for not speaking up, digging, and advocating sooner. Why didn't I trust my intuition? The still, small voice that had tried its hand at cautioning me? How could I have been so stupid? Easy. I believe that we receive our answers when we are keen to sit with their truth, knowing that it will not break us and perhaps will propel us into who we were always meant to be. We see and absorb truth when we are ready for it.

Jon's admission tore the floor from underneath me, and I struggled to know my next step. And as someone who found security in comprehending what happens next, being okay with the unknown was challenging. I had no choice but to let what I knew of our partnership crumble to the ground as if detonated. I possessed no survival tools of calculated moves to run into for shelter and away from the shrapnel. All I had was the here and now. Moment by moment. Second by second. I've found that when we feel lost, accessing our inner sanctuary will remind us precisely where repair is needed. Where was I? Heartbroken, and I would have to start right there within that heartbroken place, desolate, empty, and yet expansive.

I was trying to calculate my next move and keep myself sane while simultaneously attempting to do nothing worthy of regret. He was my person, or so I thought. I kicked Jon out and then hours later told him to come back. He shouldn't get the opportunity to shit the bed and leave me to clean it up, as far as I was concerned. By day, he watched our kids, as by that time he was working as a full-time professional touring musician and producer and could stay home as I left the house for work. At night, he slept on a friend's sofa.

While home alone, I bagged his clothes and contemplated donating them to Goodwill while imagining a scene from the film *Coming to America*. In the movie, the kids and beggars of Queens, New York, are seen wearing Prince Hakeem's royal robes after stealing them from his unattended suitcase. I imagined the same happening to Jon. I wanted him to see unexpected people on the street wearing his clothes. My final decision would be simply to throw his clothes in the dumpster, leaving him only a pair of dress shoes and a pair of swim trunks. I did all of this intentionally. I wanted the world to see how crazy he had to be to cause this amount of hurt.

In the first week, Jon called, saying, "I need to tell you everything and how I was able to do it." What else could there be? Had he not cut me enough? Emotionally bludgeoned me enough? Did I not hate him enough? Later that night, he came to the house. I got into the car and we drove to the nearest grocery store. He told me everything as we sat in the parking lot. And while this was perhaps what he needed to clear his conscience, to be free even, it had the opposite effect on me. After we arrived home and relieved the babysitter, I collapsed. My body felt heavy on the floor. I couldn't lift my arms or legs as they seemed to be pinned to the ground beneath them. I wanted to float away. Is this how it happens? I was on the verge of a nervous breakdown. I whispered "Stay" to myself, as my mind began to drift. "Stay. Stay. Stay." Jon picked me up and carried me to the bedroom. "Stay. Stay. Stay." This heaviness, this breakdown, this life, wasn't happening. According to the rules, I had done everything "right." Yet here I was on the floor on the brink of a nervous breakdown, certain that I had gotten it all wrong.

And so, life shifted. I wasn't sure what I wanted or how to proceed. I knew that I deserved more. I wasn't sure if I wanted to remain partnered. And truthfully, Jon wasn't sure if he wanted to partner with me. Keeping the partnership became less of a priority, we needed to save ourselves. We were both drowning. We were drowning in a sea of childhood traumas and adult deficits, hoping that each other (and for him another person) would fill the voids that were only reserved for our individual selves to fill.

During this time, Jon and I spent our days living in our weird partnership limbo. Jon would spend the night at a friend of our family's home, then switch with me during the day. The kids saw that Daddy slept somewhere else. I slept in what used to be our bedroom. By this time, I had given birth to our youngest sons, Jedi and Jupiter. Then only four and one year old, they were too young to know or understand that something and perhaps everything had changed. They were only babies. However, Jax, our oldest, now twelve, knew everything. His world, too, was now displaced.

As we often do when betrayed, I created a list of demands in order for us to move forward. These demands were not so I would stay but for me to even begin to engage in whatever a partnership looked like from here, be it simply co-parenting or more. The list was also written to help me feel safe. Most of my requests made sense. Some of them, not so much. During that time, Jon was expected to return to touring. I asked that he get off the road. I had many reasons for my demands. A significant part of it was fear. Fear that Jon would cause more damage or harm. And so I did what I knew to do. I hid all the "sharp objects" and scrambled for control of my environment.

The days and nights were a jumbled mess of disarray and chaos. By day I was distracted by work and day-to-day duties while we both attempted to be hands-on with our children. And by night, after the kids were in bed, I would ask question after question, trying to find answers to why Jon would choose to cause such harm. During this time, he gave me his phone to rummage through. I was in pain and grasped for anything that could comfort me. There's no poetic way to say it, but I was a wreck. I held on for dear life to Jon's phone as if it were a security blanket. His phone was the oracle to my unanswered questions. For weeks, I continued to scroll through text messages and emails, unknowingly heaping on more trauma bordering upon self-torture. If I had cultivated it, self-intimacy would have told me to stop. That this searching for more of what I already knew wasn't hurting Jon but was further harming me. And if indeed I had cultivated it, then emotional intimacy would have revealed that my need for holding on to the phone was yet another form of hiding the knives and my deep search for safety within chaos by any means necessary. I heard the passenger thoughts of our culture, reverberating in every nook and cranny of my subconscious, telling me that I was somehow at fault for Jon's unfaithfulness. If I had only done more of _____ or been more _____, this would not have happened. The passenger thoughts fed me the lie that I was the problem and Jon was an asshole who had never loved me, both of which were fallacies and irrelevant to my recovery. Both of which, if continually consumed, would lead to a juncture called nowhere. I was not the problem. I was hurting. And it didn't matter whether Jon loved me or not. The question was, to what extent did I love myself?

Do you know what's funny about fear? Fear will have you pretending and playing a game of keep-away from those you love. It will have you showing only the parts of yourself you want to see and want seen, burying the features that you consider too ugly, too dark, and somewhat unlovable. Fear will have you showing up as only half of yourself, desiring that the person sitting beside you will somehow, someway, make you whole. To show up as is within our partnerships requires vulnerability and bravery. It became apparent that Jon and I were too afraid to allow ourselves to be uncovered and fully seen.

. . . .

About two months after the revelation of Jon's infidelity, he began therapy. When Jon started therapy, I figured that if I wanted the best shot at just surviving, I should too. This was the first time in therapy for either of us. Our reason for therapy was not to see what would become of our relationship, but to save ourselves in hopes that something would become better for us as individuals. I didn't want to be swallowed up by the grief that is betrayal and infidelity.

One of the misconceptions I think many people have of treatment is that its purpose is to solve the problem. I initially wanted my therapist to fix me. I wanted her to make the trauma and the remnants thereof dissipate. I've since learned that therapy is not there to resolve but to guide you toward the answers and to serve as a mirror, reflecting the answer. My first real experience with therapy was at thirty-seven years old. I was heartbroken and figuring out my safe place in this world. My life had yet again seemed to crumble, but this time by way of my marriage. I wasn't sure what I wanted. I was angry, hurt, and in a dark place, and my friend Anxiety spiked a mile high. Nothing and no one was safe to me once again.

My therapist was a Black woman with short reddish-brown hair. In our first session, she wasn't necessarily warm and fuzzy, but she wasn't stern or rigid either. She seemed neutral, almost like an actual mirror. I shared with her how I blamed myself for not knowing that my partner was committing a betrayal of our marriage. And although I was just a child witnessing abuse first-hand, I blamed myself for not protecting my mother. I shared how I'd felt like I wasn't smart enough or good enough, or just enough. I shared how I felt paralyzed in fear sometimes and how dark and scary the world around me seemed. I explained how sometimes my mind would keep going and going, never finding a stopping place to sit and rest.

Until this point, Jon and I had made no sudden decisions. We chose not to immediately separate but instead to take each day as it came. For my divorced friends, their common regret, if any, was urgency and their need for movement while hurting. While I was upset with Jon, I was also concerned. Sure, we were now in an unknown land where we felt we barely knew each other. However, I knew him beyond the role of partner. I knew him as a friend. I was concerned about my friend, the human. And he was concerned about me too. And as a friend, I asked that he take time to seek help and figure out what he needed to be whole. Like myself, he, too, was in search of something. We were both in need of repair.

The goal was to heal the individual, and then whatever would happen would happen. We had all our cards on the table for all to see. This exposing every cave and bend of our being was our truth. The mantra: "Fuck the marriage. Save yourself." Sure, our love was real. However, love is not enough when it comes to growth within our partnerships.

And so the healing began. For me, it was a slow day-by-day drip of emotions. I had yet to start unweaving the long drawn-in knot of what had just happened. The effort it took to process what occurred in my partnership and the wounds of childhood felt all too much. I needed to fall to the floor. I needed to throw ashes, bathe in them, smearing them across the earth below. I needed to crack open, like the soil preparing itself for its seed, fully feeling it all.

CHAPTER FOUR

In the Mud

When we encounter challenging moments, we must allow ourselves the space to be "in the mud." We must grant ourselves complete agency and freedom to be frenetic, hurt, and full of rage, something I had never allowed myself to be before. Taking too much on to heal all at once is, well, too much. Slow and steady is the pace. This is lifelong work. There is no rush.

I believe that much is missed when we rush to heal too quickly. Sometimes we run into healing to absorb the pain so we don't have to feel it. We want it gone. We want to banish it into the nearest sea, never to see or experience it again. But when we rush into healing to simply quell the hurt, the symptoms, we rob ourselves of the process. And the process is everything. Our process is like water, seeping beneath our soil and into our roots.

A few weeks after I started personal therapy, Jon and I decided to begin couples therapy. We both needed a place to talk through where we were: in limbo as partners but forever co-parents. This co-parenting fact was the only guarantee of continuity. I also needed a safe space to communicate what I was feeling and experiencing with a third person qualified to act as a container between the two of us. I needed a space to yell, scream, and find my voice. I needed someone in real time to act as a vessel to hold me while I learned to use my voice and not turtle. Partnered therapy was the perfect space for discussions that were just too hard for us to have on our own.

Who were we? We were individually healing. I'm unsure if we thought we would repair the marriage through therapy, as the partnership wasn't really the focus. I think we both went into it hoping that, paired with our individual therapy, we could gather the elements of how our marriage fit into the equation of it all and how we could apply this personal work to our partnership (if at all).

IMAGO THEORY AND THE ONES WE LOVE

During one of our sessions, our therapist explained the principle of Imago Relationship Therapy, named for the Latin word for "image." Imago theory is the unintentional response to our relationships (and how we move within them), directly resulting from what we received as children or what we searched for during our youth. In other words, if you grew up lacking emotional or physical safety as a child, you will often look to your partner to provide what your parents did not. The same is true even if you received protection as a child. You will look to your partner to continue that provision within the relationship. While I am referring to romantic partnerships, this can occur within platonic relationships as well.

Often, we are unaware of operating within this space of substitution. The deeply seated desire to fill this void is rooted in our instinctive need to keep ourselves safe and survive. In other words, the love we grew up with, what we deem as recognizable, will be either what we expect to continue or what we search to replace and heal. Imago theory is a perfect example of why you may find a couple who, no matter what, will latch on to each other for dear life, even when unhealthy behavior is present. There is a search for childhood healing present that has made its way into the adult body. If you want to thrive within your partnerships, the healing of your inner child is imperative. Otherwise, the search for love and grounding in someone other than yourself will continue. Unfortunately, how this world is set up in its deficits (lack of care, mental health, and overall communal support) has produced a world full of matured bodies with childhood-induced wounds. Quite frankly, many of us do not escape childhood unscathed.

What is love
If you nurse my wound?
If you apply pressure and wrap it with silk bandages?
Love is seeing.
It is acknowledging.

Two Adult Children in Search of Security

Jon's story was not much different from mine. He, too, had childhood wounds that needed tending. He was born with an eye condition called ptosis, a congenital disability in which the eyelid muscles do not fully develop. As a result, his eyes would appear closed and required multiple surgeries. The aftermath of these surgeries ranged from your typical postsurgery stitches to more extreme shirt buttons fixed to both sides of his nose. In addition, his early school days were riddled with teasing from other children. It was a recipe for a lack of self-acceptance and self-confidence.

Unlike my story, Jon never saw his father be abusive or violent toward his mother. However, Jon did not receive much intimacy from his parents, nor did they help direct his journey toward self-awareness, which every child needs in their early development stages. You can't give what you don't have. Jon's parents were two Black people who had grown up in the segregated South. They were Black folks who worked long hours, who came from Black folks who worked from sunup to sundown. When would they have time to do this emotional work? They were just trying to keep the lights on.

My childhood was filled with hiding under tables and building a fortress of safety by turtling. His childhood was filled with fading into the black, hiding his emotions and developing barriers against external intimacy—the ability to be close to someone—since it was so lacking in his household. Both of his parents worked for the state. His father was a parole officer and his mother worked as an officer at a juvenile facility. Their job schedules caused Jon to be a latchkey kid, like many in the '80s.

He grew up knowing how to work and make ends meet when the time came to be a grown-up. But the basic life skills of intimacy and self-awareness were not present. These are lessons that our parents and caregivers teach. By second grade, he'd make himself Eggo waffles to accompany the cooked sausage his mother left on the stovetop before heading out for work. Jon would gobble down his small breakfast feast, grab his backpack, and hurry out the door. By fifth grade, this ritual would graduate to him returning home alone, where he'd make himself a snack, begin homework, or watch an episode of *Saved by the Bell* or *Ricki Lake*. His mother returned home around five o'clock, exhausted from being on her feet all day. His father returned even later. Like many families, Jon's family did the best they knew to do. No one went to bed hungry, and there was a roof over their heads; that's what mattered. However, the multitude of alone time left little space for Jon to receive guidance in cultivating self-intimacy or awareness. While one would think that the massive dose of alone time would in itself curate a sense of self-awareness, it's just not so for a young child. The adults are here to guide us into this understanding. They shape the world as we see it, molding and teaching us, whether they know it or not. And as children, we are continuously absorbing the messaging around us. This messaging creates the passenger thoughts that enter the car of life with us. Jon's parents were trying their best to provide for their son, which called for them to work long hours. But the teaching of self-awareness that parents pass down to their children wasn't readily available as a result. And Jon's parents weren't unique in this deficit. Many of our parents who grew up in or before the 1950s here in the U.S. didn't have the tools to do such self-work. Let's be honest: If you ask many people within this age demographic about therapy, self-care, and intimacy, you may be met with blank stares and dismissal. Depending on background, mental health and the freedom of self-discovery were not as easily accessible nor as prevalent as they are now. Jon's parents couldn't give him what they didn't have.

For Jon, the copious amount of alone time dispatched the message that he was his own checks and balances and that emotions were a novelty, to be shown only on after-school television shows. These messages stick to our bones and shape how we move through the world, how we see ourselves and our place in it. Jon was left alone with just his passenger thoughts and himself as the adults around him provided no guidance or resources in cultivating the tools needed to build the life he truly desired and the man he desired to be, leaving him instead to lead the life he already knew. A life of stifled feelings, devoid of vulnerability and full of secrets, a life that he was taught by the adults to replicate.

Whereas self-intimacy is our deep knowledge and connection with ourself, intentional connection is our link with others. Jon's lack of intentional connection both at home and often at school created a pathway for him to find safety only within the walls and rooms sectioned off within his mind. He made his own rules as to what was fair and proper. The rules would shift according to the set of friends or groups present. There were also moments within Jon's childhood where he witnessed dangerous acts taking place, after which there would be no conversation or check-in on his emotional state, only his returning to video games as if nothing had happened. He, too, was searching for the adults in the room to keep him safe. Jon quickly figured out that he would be accepted if he showed people only what they wanted to see.

By the time Jon and I found each other, we searched for voids to be filled. We were unaware that when we saw each other, I would see someone who could take on the job of making me "feel safe," and Jon would see someone to keep him safe within his behaviors. He placed me in the role of his mother, a space I never wanted to occupy. I was a natural nurturer, having protected those around me since I was young. When I met Jon, it was no different. Because of his trauma, he would look for chaos, while I would avoid it. While I grew up witnessing violence and abuse at the hands of my father, Jon saw risky behavior and trauma enacted within his own family. Afterward, he was left to navigate his feelings and even his fears on his own.

To Jon, I represented safety, which he would run into for shelter. We both checked each other's boxes of Imago Theory. I looked for someone to see me underneath the table, crouched down and hiding, someone who would take my hand and whisper the words that I needed to hear so many years ago: "You are protected." Jon was searching for someone who had the capacity to be present. The little boy within him craved the words "I accept you. You don't have to hide from me." Our arguments would mirror two children looking to locate security, speaking up from where our emotional development had left off. I wanted nothing more than safety. I craved it in every way imaginable. I would attempt to control everything. Jon looked for acceptance and the deep need to be fully seen, so he split himself into characters depending on who he was around and who would have him, or at least the version of himself that he felt most comfortable putting forth.

Self-intimacy is necessary to the growth and thriving of our partnerships. When we are intimate with ourselves, we are, by default, aware of our traumas, biases, and the roots of our being that may intermingle between the two. We can better communicate our needs and where it hurts when we know ourselves intimately. The emptiness that we possess is ours to heal. This healing looks different for us all. You might choose traditional talk therapy, or more alternative pathways such as psychedelic therapy or hypnotherapy. Some people find journaling super helpful to mine through the overwhelming emotions or meditation and breathwork. What have you already tried when attempting to confront old wounds or current conflicts? Was it helpful? If not, it may be time to consider other avenues toward healing. Of course, even reading this book is a tool for your continued evolution.

Our relationships are not meant to fill voids. They can only spread the salve of acknowledgment and gentleness over our bruises. I can only compare the lack of self-intimacy within a partnership to both people in a garden, pulling up flowers, leaves, roots, all in search of the weeds in the way. Both characters are aware that harm is being done to the plant, whether external or internal. Yet they don't even know where to begin. So both start pulling up everything that they see. Suppose we are not mindful of ourselves within our partnerships. In that case, we risk damaging the vital parts, the necessary components, all hoping to mitigate conflict when it arises.

Jon's and my traumas distorted our image of the present-day adults standing in the room, what love was, and how it showed up. It was impossible to show up for each other and yet neglect our own wounds. By the time we entered treatment, we were battered, bruised, and tired. Infidelity, dishonesty, and hopelessness had entered the room. Being in a relationship without dealing with childhood trauma had run its course. Jon and I, our traumas, would collide and eventually lead to our journey of self-work.

Partnering as young as we did presented its fair share of challenges. Jon felt like home, thus feeding my trauma. He was familiar. And while there were no awkward moments between us when we first met, I now recognize why that seemed to be the case. He wasn't abusive or short-tempered like my father; in fact, Jon was gentle. However, like my father, he could be emotionally vacant and possess a deep-seated pull toward chaos. For Jon, the infidelity was not the only culprit, the secrets were too. Keeping secrets while maintaining an illusion of a perfect home and managing what could be an otherwise peaceful life is chaotic. While on the road, he would seek risk. He'd find himself in crowded bars, meeting up with strangers to "go party," experimenting with cocaine, molly, and always cannabis. If there was a risk that could scratch his itch for dopamine, he wanted to be a part of it. What was done on the road stayed on the road. After Jon disclosed everything, I would imagine the call that I could have gotten from his fellow bandmate telling me that he had passed away from an overdose or some secret that I'd yet to be made aware of. I imagined the denial that would flood my system and having to tell our children. This thought would make me so very angry. Angry at Jon, his father who also lived a life of infidelity, and all of those who knew Jon's hidden side and watched with hands tied. I hated them all. How far could he pass the boundary of almost getting caught, crashing and burning, while surviving it all by the skin of his teeth? That was the life and chaos he chased. I was familiar with this personality and manifestation of trauma. Managing it felt like home.

I was too young to be aware of who I was on my own. This unearthing is a task that we all must do in early adulthood. Partnering with oneself first is the obstacle that many have difficulty achieving. Let's face it, it is hard. Really, who wants to dig through their childhood trauma and only look within to heal? It makes sense that it would be so much easier to partner with those around us, ask (and sometimes even demand) that they heal us, kiss our wounds, and make it better, only to find out that that is just not possible.

It All Comes Back to You

Self-intimacy is the pathway to connection for all of our relationships. We must recognize what exactly is hurting and do our own work. As long as I expected Jon to show up and be the father that I needed as a child (again, referencing the Imago Theory), he would always fail, and I would stay stuck as that scared little girl, terrified of the thunder. As long as Jon expected me to show up as the present parent to keep him safe and responsible, I would always fail, and he would stay stuck as the little boy, crying out for acceptance and seeking chaos. We had to both make space and begin on our adventure. When I stopped looking at Jon as my father, I could genuinely see him as my partner.

Being in relationship requires an expansion in love toward others and ourselves and an awareness of where the two connect.

During our introduction, I spoke of a door. The pathway on which we meet ourself during labor's transition. Whether by therapy or other resources, doing the work *is* the door. The follow-through and exercising of the tools gained is kindred to the transition. It is a labor of love for certain, but worth the work in order to move from simply surviving to thriving within our partnerships.

Being in partnership is one of life's greatest labors, and yet it yields one of life's greatest rewards. I remember our therapist mentioning that partnership is a continual selfless act, requiring you to listen, hear, and understand another's perspective. Much like labor, partnership in any form is a great teacher, calling us to deeply reflect and, if we are open to it, grow. Usually, our partner is the opposite of us in some way. They carry their gifts, abilities, and socioemotional intelligence. Being in partnership requires that we live in constant awareness that another perspective, story, and journey are sitting across from us. That there may be unresolved trauma and apparent triggers.

Fun fact: I believe that most couples do not see their partners as people but simply as extensions of themselves. I think that somewhere in the notion that "the two become one," there is a bit lost in translation. While two people become "one" in uniting for the partnership's common goal, two people still exist, holding two individual journeys to the present day. Two ways of thinking are active. To heal myself from the hurt of betrayal and begin cultivating my first relationship (with myself), I had to detach from Jon, peeling away the layers by which we had become molded and meshed together. I had to see myself as an individual first to stand a chance at seeing Jon, even if as only a co-parent. If we acknowledge and celebrate our distinct paths, there is so much room for growth and grace when these aspects are uplifted, seen, and allowed to show up as is.

Have you ever been in a disagreement with a partner or friend? One in which there's quite a bit of back-and-forth, and no matter what is said, you both seem to hit a wall? I mean, it's a stalemate. Perhaps, no matter how you explain your point and the words in which you frame it, the words don't seem to penetrate. Maybe it also appears that you or your partner feels an internal wall. You feel emotionally stuck.

When this happens, I first encourage folks to look inward. Ask yourself, "What do I hear versus what am I understanding?" So often, we listen with the anticipation of responding instead of giving space for both people within the conversation to be present and desiring resolution or simply understanding, permitting ourselves to hear the other person's words. Then and only then can we allow ourselves a pathway of comprehending their unique viewpoint.

Second, ask yourself who is doing the listening. Are you listening from your adult self or your child self? The tricky thing about our childhood experiences is that many of our feelings, the parts that feel tender and sore, are birthed from our upbringing and carried into our relationships. The same is true if you had a positive upbringing. For example, one parent may have worked outside the home while the other cared for the children and prepared meals. Now, as an adult, how you view nurturing and provision is likely designated to one person or even specific gender norms. Perhaps your partner's nurturing style is different from your parents', but it is still present.

How Imago Theory applies to relationships:

- An example would be saying "You are never there for me" during the conflict, and the truth is, of course, that they are there for you. However, within that moment, past emotions of being a young child and feeling as if your parent or caregiver was "never there for you" are triggered within the conversation. This example is why it is imperative that one quickly take a breath and a moment to evaluate whether their child self is in the driver's seat of the disagreement or misunderstanding. Distinguishing between the two is vital for proper understanding and reaching a place of clarity. Once we check in for a bit, the door opens for conversation expansion.

Checking in looks like:

- Repeat to yourself what you hear your partner/friend/colleague saying. What is the message being heard? Example: "You are never there for me."
- Be curious if the message you are hearing is a common theme or a sore spot that comes up for you in this relationship and others. Everyone can't be conspiring against us, using the same tools. This could indicate that our childhood selves may be listening in and communicating.
- Where is the defense located? In the example given above, perhaps you think that those in your life are "never" there for you. Ask yourself, "Is this an area that needed care when I was a child? Was I deficient in this need being met?" Now ground yourself in the present, and ask, "Does this sensation feel familiar?"

Checking in grants an opportunity for self-gentleness and for your partner to show up as your partner, not filling the deficit left by your childhood wound but rather spreading a salve of acknowledgment and "seeing" over it. In other words, when we realize that the disagreement isn't about carrots but cars, we can step back and begin having a dialogue about vehicles instead of two people having two different conversations. If, after checking in, partners recognize that perhaps one of them or both are speaking from childhood wounds, each can take turns expressing what's coming up for them. One person shares, while the other acts as a container, listens, and holds space. Doing this creates a level of intimacy between both people that declares and affirms each other's safety.

Remember the analogy of becoming sanctuary to ourselves? The same holds when it comes to our partnerships. We can offer a safe space for our partners to lay their heads when we are a sanctuary.

IDOLS IN LOVE'S TEMPLE

When studying Greece's old temples, we find that having a sanctuary was vital for one's communion with God. The same is true when we look at Egypt's ancient temple structure as well as Rome's, and even present-day churches'. These communal benchmarks within our societies provided a space for direct dialogue with God. The same is true within our relationships. Being in an alliance affords us all an opportunity to connect with our higher power, and more specifically, our highest selves. When we are asked to consider another's perspective, this is our chance to become more _____-like than we were before.

Listening to understand produces the same result. I believe that many relationships view disagreement as disharmony. It is not. It is simply an opportunity to learn more, not only about our partner but ourself. When we operate from being a sanctuary to our partner, family member, or friend, we can access our inner teacher to guide us with curiosity and light instead of simply making our point during the conflict. When emotionally activated, we can check in and be curious about what's coming up. If you are the person who feels triggered, ask for space, tap into that still, small voice, and ask, "What's coming up for me?" If you notice something coming up for your partner, you can offer, "Hey, I noticed that you became quiet. May I ask, what's coming up for you?" Like the ancient temples holding space and holy prayers, this awareness allows for a coordinated response in relationships.

Sanctuary is also a place of refuge and safety. We stand as living, breathing sanctuaries for ourselves and one another. It is the humane protection of our collective wellness and care. As mentioned, we are all looking for safe spaces for our thoughts, words, and emotions to locate a protected place to lay our heads. What if we shifted our thinking from "I am right" to "I am trying to find sanctuary for my thoughts, and emotional space around the issue presented." What if we viewed one another in that way? When we are expressing our truth, that's what we are doing. We are searching for sanctuary and solace in putting the kerfuffle to rest. We are looking to be seen and heard.

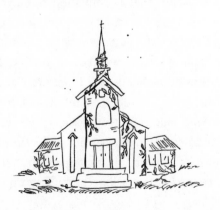

How do my partner and I become a sanctuary for each other? We must first remove the ego. It's the mud in an otherwise clean temple. I know. Either it's easier said than done, or you don't have an ego. Here's the liberating truth: We all have an ego. It's always there, reminding us of our self-importance, which is neither good nor bad. However, it's not needed when becoming a sanctuary for each other. I like to think of ego as the weeds. Ego often gets in the way and prohibits our growth and our nourishment. Much like the weeds that plague our outdoor garden, our ego possesses the power to cut off our ability to provide our partner with deep and rich soul food and essential awareness, and it prohibits our receiving of love, reciprocity, and intimacy. When our ego is present, so is self-preservation and the preservation of being "right." We can neither give nor receive when the weeds of our ego are present. And in the words of my dear friend Melanie Fiona, "Do you want to be right? Or do you want to be well?"

There is empathy and patience to be had for our ego as well. Within our sanctuary, the ego can serve as an idol that we have built as a form of protection. Laying aside our ego and allowing our partner's truth to permeate by actively listening is a form of vulnerability. For me, releasing ego required that I remove the idea that my way of seeing the world was the "right way," instead of simply my way, and that it contained room for fallacy and therefore improvement. I would gather the world into groups of good or bad, safe or unsafe, and as those to either be pulled in or fully avoided. Pulling up the weeds of ego looked like holding between the palms of my hands that I mattered, and that despite his past, Jon mattered as well. The moment I could scrap the belief that only *my* pain, *my* healing, and *my* trauma mattered was when I could see Jon fully in his. Releasing ego may feel sacrificial, almost as if we are offering up our fatted calf. Perhaps even painful. However, much like the pulling up of weeds, it is necessary, as it is the very thing that chokes progress within our partnerships.

We must allow our higher selves to take place and say: *Although it is human, ego is not welcome here.* Only then are we able to see and take invariant perspectives. Within the partnership, we need to feel that our words, feelings, and thoughts will not stay homeless, searching for a safe space to land. When we demonstrate tangible care and active listening, we begin to thrive within our partnership instead of simply making our point. Sowing seeds of intentional listening will produce a legacy of trust and safety.

Allow me to give you an example from nature. Have you ever looked at the pattern of trees? Although their massive trunks reach high, resembling the skyscrapers of the city, there is a pattern revealed between their branches of leaves. Through their leaves, sunlight peeks through, offering a chance at photosynthesis and growth. This consideration is not by accident but in fact by design. The botanist Dr. Tanisha Williams shared the story of tree canopy cooperation, also known as tree architecture. These trees have a secret. Their branches grow and spread in an orchestrated fashion, allowing enough light for the surrounding trees. They disperse their leaves, twisting their earthen bodies, working together so that each tree gets its needs met. They recognize that there is enough sun for us all.

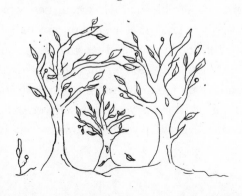

To thrive within our partnership, we must fight well together. There will be moments of disagreement. It is inevitable. And in the case where there are never arguments, trust me, someone is lying. The focus should be on disagreeing well, not avoiding disputes altogether. You have two relationships. In one, the partners fight endlessly. They disagree on everything from the curtains to the grocery list. They collide and quarrel about possible school choices and where the unfolded laundry belongs. And then you have another relationship in which the partners never fight, and they avoid conflict at all costs. Things seem like smooth sailing, yet a storm of unsaid words and disrupted truth is brewing underneath it all. Which relationship is better? Neither. Both reside on the struggle boat of relationships. One couple keeps their words buried at sea, while the other unleashes them without reserve. The answer is not avoiding conflict but learning how to move within it.

RULES OF ENGAGEMENT

This wellness within our discourse often starts with setting rules of engagement. For example, write down a few things that feel like "flooders." Flooders are statements that will breach the dam of harm and, by default, cause shutdown. Try to keep the list to two to three nonstarters. Talk through these things with each other, being vulnerable in their origin and why. Treat those things as the holy grail of conversation crushers from then on. An example of flooders would be using exaggerated terms like "always" and "never." In fact, no one ever "alwayses" or "nevers." We humans are far too inconsistent to perform such a feat. Another example of a flooder would be using verbal finger pointing. Using external terms like "you" to highlight what you feel on the

inside is usually a nonstarter. Examples: Because of you, I
_____. You made me _____. You always/never _____.

Using such language in any setting—partnership, platonic, or
professional—tends to immediately put people on defense. If
the goal is to be heard and understood, let us make it easy. And
while that ease may require vulnerability, transparency, and perhaps even fearlessness from us, employing these communication
tools is one of the most efficient ways of sharing how we feel and
being understood.

Another example of a flooder can be discussing what is irrelevant to the discussion or area of disconnect. I found that when
we intentionally center on the actual break within the relationship and the agreed-upon path forward, this acts as a guardrail.
Give this approach a try: "I feel _____." "When _____
happened, I felt _____."

Another rule of engagement is the commitment to be conscious
of our words. This awareness looks like speaking our truth,
joined with the responsibility of not intentionally harming the
other person with our words. When I feel that my emotions may
cause the dam of harsh words to break, I will commit to taking a
moment for myself. I've heard that some relationships use safe
words when the expressions escape within the pitch black of
emotions. Some say "Take five."

A final example of fighting well is grounding by way of sen-
sory. When things feel escalated, use your senses for grounding.
Touch each other. A quick hand-to-hand touch can do wonders.
If you are a person who sees, keep eye contact. When we begin
looking off, perhaps into our phone or out the window, or isolate
ourselves, refraining from touching of self or partner, we block

off two of the most important senses that remind us that we are in the here and now. By cutting off our senses, we can then venture back into the spaces where we felt rejected or neglected and the rooms where we felt lost and alone. Our inner child can then begin to drive but not control the adult conversation. By simply keeping eye contact, fixing our ears to our partner's words or the rustling wind, or a quick touch on the hand, we are reminded that we are no longer experiencing the past, but indeed the present.

Jon and I went from a partnership full of invisible wounds to what we like to call a treehouse partnership. This treehouse that Jon and I have built has taken time and work. But I'll never forget the culmination of days, weeks, months when it finally hit us that our child selves had been conversing for quite some time. Imagine two adult bodies, but yet children. For the first time, we indeed saw each other. We began to see the small childlike parts screaming out for those things that were lacking. And we started to speak to and up for those parts. Jon began seeing his child self, trying to find acceptance and his place. He would share when those parts that had been buried beneath the soil made their way to the surface. I would begin to talk to those parts in response, affirming my acceptance. That I loved him . . . all of him. That I forgave him. I discovered child Brandi searching for protection and safety in our treehouse from a chaotic world. And when my child wounds would make their presence known, Jon would begin speaking to those parts in response—affirming my safety. When we see our child selves, we can operate with empathy. And this opens the door.

We humans need cover beyond physical buildings. How cool would it be if we began to see ourselves as the old sanctuaries of yesterday where people would find refuge from the storms of life? How amazing would it be in return if we knew that when navigating challenging moments, we could find safety within the temple sitting across from us, knowing that our feelings and words are safe and no longer lost?

Jon and I are safe and protected within our treehouse. We are high above the ground within our natural bungalow where no one, including our past traumas, can sever the branches, creating a sanctuary for the two of us. Within our treehouse, there is a refuge for seven-year-old Brandi and Jon. There is love and acknowledgment. There is no need for turtling, as we have made room for us both within the protection of each other.

Much like the birthing mother I spoke of earlier, we are all birthing something within our relationships. What do you hope to birth within yours? How do we thrive within our collaboration? First, we reimagine and re-form our beginnings. We create sanctuaries and safe spaces. We remove the idols of ego and tap into our higher selves to create safety. We acknowledge that although two may become one, there is still an individual perhaps buried beneath the covering of their life's adventure, past, and childhood.

We value each other, knowing that we benefit from each other's thriving existence and awareness of self, much like the trees. We need each other, and we need ourselves.

• •

FOR REFLECTION

What are the passenger thoughts surrounding partnerships you've picked up along the way?
Do you recognize elements of Imago Theory being played

out within your relationships (not limited to romantic partnerships)?

What is your fighting style? Do you fight well?

How does ego (the weeds) show up in your relationships?

Identify your relational flooders.

CHAPTER FIVE

Reparenting Ourselves

W hen I found out that I was pregnant with my eldest son, Jax, I was in complete denial. I was almost two weeks late, and at the time—just months into my marriage and the ripe age of twenty-four—one of the things that I could rely on was my monthly confidante, my period, to make its arrival the exact same day each month. This particular month, she didn't come, and I still thought it had to be something else. We had been so cautious. We wanted to wait until we were more settled before starting our family.

I remember peeing on the stick and thinking that perhaps I was just late, and my pregnancy was all in my head. I was sure the result would be negative. Sure, I was drained and went to bed around eight each night due to exhaustion. Of course, my appetite had increased to that of an NFL linebacker. I checked all the boxes for pregnancy symptoms. However, the force of denial was strong with this one. I was scared. I wasn't ready. I'd hoped to navigate this new adventure of being somebody's wife a bit longer before settling into the role of mother. Becoming a parent felt all too soon and too fast. However, I remember also feeling that it would be okay and that we would be okay. I peed on the stick and the two lines stared back at me. So would begin our parenting journey.

Back then, I was a musician, performing and playing shows, coupled with late-night rehearsals at makeshift studios and storage rooms turned practice spaces. I imagined a few more years of getting to know myself as an artist, cultivating my songwriting craft while making my way through Nashville writer's rounds before entering the role of mother. I was acutely aware of the shift that having a child within that time and space could create in my early twenties. I remember being somewhat afraid to share that I was pregnant out of fear of being left out, as I would be the first of my friends to have kids. Now that I was pregnant, I feared being viewed as different, not the same hungry, gritty, and, most important, creatively available musician as before. There was fear that folks would assume that I was too tired or too pregnant to perform, or write, or do whatever it was that I did before my secret made its way aboveground. I was also afraid that friends would stop including me within their twentysomethings revelry. Granted, I was a bit of a homebody and enjoyed a quiet and early turndown. However, the choice whether to go out or not was mine and mine alone. I reached for the fragments of myself that I knew would dissipate into the well of "before motherhood." I was married and now pregnant in my early twenties, and I believe a part of me grieved for the freedom that being carefree and so very young afforded. I was now going to be somebody's mama. Exploring my early twenties would have to continue with a baby in tow.

When I became pregnant, my desire was to be accepted still, valid still, as opposed to discarded as no longer useful. I desperately wished that no matter the stage of life I was in, I would still be welcomed and received. Looking back, this was a unique opportunity to reparent and give myself the acceptance, assurance, and validation I desperately needed.

Reparenting is the act of nurturing and attending to yourself as a loving parent would. It is loving your current and child self that may be screaming out for more softness and gentleness in a way that is so very unique and intentional. My life had shifted quicker at that moment than I had hoped. My twenties would be filled with dirty diapers and playground sand, unlike the exploration and freedom many of my peers were experiencing. Radical acceptance at that time would be acknowledging that while my life would now look different, it was still my life and mine for the making. It was still grand, perhaps even beautiful.

After eighteen hours of labor, the nurse placed my son, Jax, on my chest. A million stares seemed to surround me. I felt awkward in my new role as a mother. I immediately sensed pressure to feel an overwhelming capacity for joy and love. During my pregnancy, I watched videos of pregnant people giving birth with tears streaming down their face because the privilege of doing so was just that beautiful. I wanted to be them. I wanted to feel that, or to express my feelings in that way. Instead, there were no tears or sobbing for the bright light that had entered the world. Instead, there was just awe. It was as if my heart had whispered a prayer in the stillness of the night, and birthing Jax was the manifestation of those unknown prayers made known. It was like rising before dawn and having the opportunity to witness the sunrise and acknowledging the awe within the fact that the sun that rises and sets in Tennessee is the same sun that makes its appearance over the Sahara. I felt this same awe within my body. There was no room for tears within the moment, only the deep exhale of breath as life had entered the tiny hospital room and my heart. There were no tears of exhilaration like the mamas in the videos I watched. There was simply calm, and this was just as divine for me. I can only equate it to the sigh that a parishioner gives after uttering the word "Amen." Within that Amen, the awkwardness that I initially felt quickly faded into the background of the hospital room.

My postpartum season was a haze. I felt pressure to be and do more. I remember feeling the need to keep up and that if I didn't, my identity would get lost within the shuffle of motherhood. Back then, the clock told me that I hadn't accomplished enough to rest within this new identity of motherhood and that I had to hustle and hustle hard. There was no resting for my postpartum body. My rest and reprieve would have to be earned. Jon's mom came to help and support us, offering to do our laundry or anything that needed to be done around the house. I declined her offers and instead opted to move my postpartum body around the house, bleeding and sore. I had something to prove to the world and my mother-in-law. I wanted the world to know that I was worthy of my rest and parenting. I wanted to do it right, and at that moment, "doing it right" meant folding my own damn underwear, vacuuming, and nurturing my son and those around me. I wanted to prove that I could do it all.

Looking back, I believe that I suffered from undiagnosed postpartum anxiety, a postnatal mental illness that often goes unrecognized. Postnatal anxiety is often viewed as simply a nervous first-time parent when it is much more. This disorder triggers feelings of constant worry and hypervigilance. For me, it showed up as this never-ending checklist in my mind. Did I throw away the dirty diaper? Did I put away anything that could be a hazard? And almost everything felt like a hazard—the dirty diaper left on the changing table, the changing table itself, and so much more. I would meditate on the what-ifs and immerse myself in thoughts of prevention. If Jax was crying, I would rush in with dread and anxiety, preparing myself just in case something was wrong. My postpartum anxiety showed up as overextended awareness and stress. There would be days when I would experience alternating ruminations of mothering "the right way" and of worst-case scenarios. My heart would race as I experienced panic attacks while keeping up with my safety checklist. Like most birthing folks who wrestle with anxiety pre-baby, motherhood kicked the anxiety into high gear.

Postpartum anxiety also kicked my survival tools into high gear. Most of what I felt was due to post-baby hormones. Much of it was also tied to my wound and need for safety by way of control. Postpartum and all that comes with birthing a baby felt unruly. Babies themselves are uncontrollable. And like many who have dealt with trauma, the idea of this type of rebellion terrified me.

Along with the postpartum anxiety, FOMO (fear of missing out) played a high tune in my mind. Jax was born the week before Thanksgiving. I decided to pack our car and go visit family for the holidays. I wanted our family to meet our new addition. I wanted to be around love and home. And so I headed south on a road trip six days postpartum. My breasts were full of milk, and I was still bleeding from birth.

There was no such thing as Instagram in 2006 or an online group to reach out to for postpartum support, especially regarding the struggle of breastfeeding. My mother didn't breastfeed; neither did Jon's. There was no one to turn to, and if there is one thing that breastfeeding calls for, it's a village of support, whether online or in real life. I had previously called the lactation consultant from the hospital to ask what to do after explaining the challenges I was having nursing Jax and how engorged my breasts were. She provided me with two options: to continue or end my breastfeeding journey. These were the obvious choices. I was honestly hoping that she would give me a plan C. It all seemed too stressful to add to the first-time jitters as a new parent and the brewing of postpartum anxiety. I was alone and in desperate need of support after five days of trying and trying and more people telling me that "it didn't take all that" than actually supporting me in this time. I stopped breastfeeding. As I shared with the lactation consultant, she quickly explained how to dry up my milk instead of simply providing a bit of guidance into what my body was doing. I took her recommendation. Before we headed south, I wrapped my breasts in cabbage leaves and took Sudafed in hopes of drying up my milk.

Jon and I rode in the car with our newborn; my engorged cabbage-wrapped breasts leaked as we listened to the radio. My fear of being enough presented itself within our car ride. I was anxious. Would I appear motherly enough? Had I remembered to pack everything in our overnight bag? I hoped to appear so much wiser, smarter, and stronger. My bones ached and my spirit felt the weight of the exhaust as the bumps and highway potholes kneaded into my body. Upon our arrival at my parents' house, I knew I had perhaps not made the best decision. Everything was too overwhelming, too loud, and too much for my postpartum self. Sure, with our family, as expected, love was present. However, I was a wreck. I remember my parents, Jon, and I standing in our bedroom talking and catching up, only for them to leave the room and the dam of tears burst forth as if I had been holding them from breaching. It was all too much, too many opinions, and too much stress. I felt the need to perform within the environment instead of what my postpartum body needed to do, just rest. I had been masking the inner frenzy and upheaval that I had been experiencing. I'd smiled and laughed, affirming that I was okay when I was on the verge of collapsing under the pressure of it all.

If I had accessed the teacher within, if I had been present to parent myself in the moment, I more than likely would have heard "Rest" resounding loudly and "Stay your ass at home." On my first go at postpartum with my first child, I wasn't aware that rest was what my body needed, so it would make sense that I drove to see family six days after giving birth. I didn't know but quickly realized what my body needed. This wasn't it.

Shame also made its way to the surface. Giving birth was supposedly one of the most ordinary and natural things that humans experience. And here I was struggling. I was struggling to obtain sleep and everyday normalcy. Struggling to make peace with the newly formed chaos and unpredictability within the scope of being a new parent. Why was this so hard for me yet appeared so effortless for others? There was so much that I didn't know and had yet to discover and unlock within myself. I feared being unequipped, and for that, I was ashamed.

REPARENTING AND TENDING

As a new parent, I had not yet discovered how to walk in my role as a mother. However, one thing was sure: Whether I had ever chosen to become a mother or not, I needed to learn to reparent *myself* alongside this new adventure. Like branches propagated from their mother plant, we all come from somebody. And while sometimes those parent plants spring forth from nurturing and nutrient-dense soil, many of us come from those who did the best they could with whatever grounding they possessed. And because of this, for us to thrive, we must learn how to reparent ourselves, no matter how divine or sovereign our roots may flow.

I define reparenting not necessarily as a redo or a wiping of the slate, as there are just some things within our childhood that we will never be able to "redo" or erase, but more as parenting ourselves *again,* in this moment, where we are now. Reparenting involves giving ourselves unconditional love, grace, and mindfulness that we are learning, evolving, and growing, the way we did as a child. It is becoming the parental figure we need now for ourselves.

Reparenting is for everyone and not just those with less than ideal or traumatic childhoods. As mentioned, to reparent is not to redo or undo anything. Reparenting is a tool we must put into practice to thrive. As we are constantly growing and learning, we are also unlearning the patterns that no longer align with who we are today as adults. What are the ways of thinking (not necessarily negative) that served you well at one point in your life but are no longer helpful or even practical? Recognizing these areas will require you to parent (guide/grow) yourself into a new, better approach. As long as we are growing, we must reparent ourselves in every season. Reparenting allows us to mother and father ourselves and to handle ourselves more gently, as a loving parent would.

The first step of reparenting involves emotional provision. Ask your current self, "What are you seeking?" More often than not, the thing we seek acts as a compass helping us locate our needs. Our fears may also reveal our needs. Is it validation, acceptance, approval, love? More than likely, if all roads lead to these needs, your inner child and current self may be foraging. Much like our inner child, our adult selves need love and support too. And who better to offer it than us? Who better than you to reassure yourself, as a parent would a restless child?

Reparenting looks like the erasure of the clock. As a doula, one of the many questions I receive is about milestones. "When will my baby start sleeping through the night? When will they start walking? Is this normal according to the manmade timeline?" If we are honest, many parents absorb the answer, be it yes or no, as the litmus test for whether they are doing it right. Many of our parents were no different. And how we moved and grew through this world was metabolized as a direct result of their parenting and a test of whether *they* were doing it right, whether they were normal. A significant portion of reparenting ourselves is letting go of our imaginary timelines. Our life is like water and requires the constant flow of a sea captain navigating its waves. So, you wanted to be _____ by this time. You wanted to be further along in _____ by now. Is this *your* timeline? *Your* milestone? Or is it someone else's that has now become enmeshed within your own? Release expectations that either no longer or perhaps never mattered to *you*. They only prohibit you from discovering *your* path.

REPARENTING OURSELVES FROM A PLACE OF EMPATHY

I want you to know that whether we are birthing tiny humans or dreams and visions, especially when working with anyone outside ourself, there will always be components outside our control. This fact alone can kick-start a need to regain our footing or move into high gear, sparking our survival as opposed to thriving. Whether you just birthed your dream or an actual child, you may feel an overload of anxiety, a deep-rooted fear of letdown now that it is out in the world. Give yourself the gift of patience, empathy, and the allowance of failure. Yes, failure. A parent who observes their child walking for the first time and, of course, falling doesn't judge or dismiss their little one's attempt at finding their footing and next steps across the living room floor. They cheer them on to the next. In our reparenting, we must offer ourselves the same gifts, self-empathy and encouragement.

Try not to punish yourself over what you don't (or didn't) know. Reparenting ourselves requires that we remove punishment as a tool for comprehension or course correction. I can offer to you now that this pathway of development is maladaptive and has never steered us toward our highest good. I get it. Shame and being sat in the corner of our classroom may have been the means used toward us during our youth to spawn self-reflection. However, if we are honest, it didn't work then either. As children, it taught us that within our learning and figuring it out, we are not worthy of kindness and love, but instead isolation and deprivation. So now that we are adults, what do we offer ourselves when we are "doing it wrong," not performing up to par, or our milestones present differently from our peers? We deliver shame as a tool for remedy. We deprive ourselves of the empathy and love needed in that learning space. How do we reparent ourselves when feeling shame? We present ourselves as a holy offering of patience, and with patience comes tremendous and radical tenderness. This self-devotion sounds like "You are doing your best." "You knew what you knew, and now you know better."

For me after birthing our son, its sound echoed, "Your right to post-birth healing and self-compassion is not something to be earned or rewarded. It is yours." And to that, I offer the same to you. After birthing—and I'm talking about any kind of birthing, not just a child—you do not have to earn your way to self-kindness or gentleness. Softness is yours and must be claimed.

SIGNS THAT REPARENTING IS NEEDED

When is reparenting necessary? What are the signs that we need to reparent ourselves?

We reparent ourselves during moments of activation and triggers. When we feel heated and triggers from our past make their way home within our present, and even during moments that some may view as our failures, this is a moment for reparenting.

Start by sitting. I like to implement a physical component within my self-parenting practice. I grab my hand and visualize it as the hand of my younger self, which may be feeling frenzied. I imagine sitting with her as the adult in the room. I remind her that all is well. And that if it's not, it will be. That I'm here for us both. Then, while still holding my hand, I shift my focus to my current self and imagine holding my adult self's hand at that moment. I consider who I am now. And I sit there as if I were a loving parent, just witnessing how far I've come. Like a parent, I tell myself how wonderful and beautiful I am, even in this challenging moment. I tell myself that this trigger, this harrowing day, this moment, doesn't define me. That I'm human and have a right to be so. I remind myself how loved I am even now.

Reparenting is needed when we hit a wall. When we feel frustrated that what worked for us before is no longer working now, be it with work, creatively, interpersonally, or otherwise. Sometimes, even as adults, we yearn for permission. So, in these moments, give it. Give yourself permission to let go of the old ways, titles, and parts that feel stagnant. Maybe you used to find your most inspiring and creative juices flowed at night. Because of schedule, age, and life's ever-evolving shifts, nights might feel now like a nonstarter regarding your creative flow. I want you to know that you don't have to stay here. You can evaluate what worked and no longer does and give yourself permission to shift. Give yourself permission to change, release, and even outgrow.

This may sound obvious. However, when our fundamental needs (rest, nourishment, care) feel nonexistent and ignored, this may be a sign of a need to parent ourselves. While one can absolutely run on empty, one can do so for only a short time. It wouldn't be until the birth of my youngest son, Jupiter, that I learned how to truly mother myself. When I gave birth to Jax, my mother was still alive. By the time I had Jedi and Jupiter, I would have to navigate my mothering journey without a maternal figure in my life. Not having my mother present revealed a door of opportunity to explore how I needed mothering. When I was tired and overextended, I would pause and check in, asking what I needed, as if I were a mother, caring for myself from a maternal point of view. The maternal or paternal instinct would reveal my soul's longing for a nap upon checking in.

Being motherless while mothering prioritized mothering myself, a task I hadn't had to perform with my oldest child. When you are unusually short-tempered, and your feelings seem to sit on your skin like dew, it's a clear indicator that there may be a need to take a step back and assess. Of what can I let go? What am I striving to prove? Where can I slow down a bit? What is not needed? Like a parent, offering the gift of reparenting ourselves will allow us to pay attention to those needs when they seem out of balance and neglected. We must tend to thrive.

Just Checking In

Years later, I would learn the power that checking in provided. One of the most valuable reparenting tools I have acquired is the ability of checking in with myself. Perhaps as a child, you didn't receive this type of nurturing from the adults in your life. Maybe no one asked how something made you feel; instead, there was a sense of urgency to simply carry on. Don't feel it, simply deal with it, scour it clean so no one witnesses its detritus. And so now, as grown-ups, we do just that. We carry on. We were never taught to be with ourselves. And this is not to be confused with being simply *by* ourselves. There is a difference. Growing up, we sat in the corner of our classrooms or were sent to our bedroom after misbehaving. The messaging sent and eventual passenger thought received was that being with ourselves was and is punishment. And why would you ever check in with someone you were forced to visit under these conditions? It's no wonder there are so many adults who struggle with checking in.

If this mirrors your experience growing up, we must unlearn how we view sitting with ourselves. How? It's a practice. It's a ritual. It is perhaps an underworked muscle knowing that we are the adults now and genuinely want what's best for us. It all starts with inquisitiveness and maybe asking ourselves the questions that the adults in our lives didn't know or have the tools to ask. The million-dollar question is "Are you okay?" I wholeheartedly believe that you deserve to have *you* in your corner.

Like any relationship you check in with, you become more aware of and gentler toward yourself. If you know that you have been hard-pressed to meet expectations, your patience toward yourself and others waxes thin between the ripples of overextending and complete depletion. When we practice checking in, we can reparent ourselves and give our current selves precisely what we need instead of simply requiring that we push through, perform, and meet said expectations despite our limits, intuition, and perhaps even boundaries. When we check in, we acknowledge that we are worthy of acceptance still. That we are humans healing still.

· · · · · · · · · ·

When we parent ourselves, the still, small voice calls out our spirit's importance. In our society, the peer pressure of perfection, success, and all the things we think we need to prove our worth tell us that we must do just that. Prove. Constantly prove, earn, and strive for what is already ours: approval, acceptance, love, and a necessity for our universal presence here on this earth. Pausing right now, what would your internal parent tell you about yourself? What has it noticed about the way you're currently moving through the world? What would your internal parent recommend in love?

For me, my reparenting or internal mothering reminds me that I am important and I am enough. It affirms that for me to nurture those around me, I must first nurture myself. I must do so without regret or exemption of worthiness. Self-nurturing is the key to thriving while parenting and also while simply moving through this journey called life.

Life and Weaning

One thing I know for sure is that our reparenting evolves and changes. I believe that many of us try our hand at keeping the normalcy and rhythm of prior parenting to no avail. We go from birthing our physical and spiritual babes to nurturing and showing them how to navigate the world around them. I'll never forget the weaning of Jupiter, my youngest and last baby. I knew it was time. My body felt it. However, my heart was breaking in two. I had been either pregnant or nursing for seven years straight by this time. There were no breaks between the two chasms of carrying life and nourishing it. I was first pregnant with Jedi, then breastfed Jedi, became pregnant with Jupiter, then breastfed Jupiter. This song and dance lasted a whole seven years. I fought the thought of weaning, although I knew that eventually it would come. Truthfully, I hoped that Jupiter would wean on his own and that it would be a clean break instead of the shattering feeling of bone tearing away from its marrow.

I would make up all the reasons to continue. "What if one of our little ones catches a cold?" Breast milk is like a magical elixir, and while providing it I felt like a magical unicorn or some prophet who could heal. I also knew that breastfeeding is good for the birthing person, significantly reducing ovarian and breast cancer chances. The longer a person breastfeeds, the more their percentages decrease for developing these diseases and others such as diabetes. I also grappled with the idea of weaning, as this was my last baby. After weaning, I would never breastfeed a baby again. I held on. I conjured reason upon reason to keep going. However, I knew and felt that weaning was what my body needed. It had been so long since my body had been my own. I had been tethered to a tiny human for several years in some way, shape, or form. By this point, every move I made was connected to how it would affect the baby growing inside or the baby I nurtured outside. I had begun to crack open at the seams, which is how I knew it was time to shift. Parenting myself in this moment meant not ignoring the cracking I was witnessing within myself. We try to ignore what we know to be true about our bodies or emotional states in hopes that if we wade a little longer, try a little harder, and perhaps dig a little deeper, the tide will turn, and no decision will need to be made. But when actively parenting oneself, it's clearer to see when we must take action and not simply float at sea barely staying above the water.

Crack
Break
Expand
It's all a shift

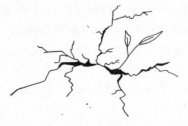

It's all necessary
It's all an opportunity for growth.

Jon and I decided to take a road trip. I hoped to take the weekend to begin drying up my milk. I knew that it would take a while and for sure longer than two or three days. However, I knew that to begin, I needed to take space away. Weaning Jedi, my middle child, was a lot easier. We had endured the late eves of night weaning. By the time I decided to wean him, I had already significantly reduced my breastfeeding to only once a day. I was also pregnant with Jupiter, so my milk had also decreased. I received the positive pregnancy test and made the active decision to stop breastfeeding Jedi. Simple enough. With Jupiter, it was a bit complicated. There were stops and starts to our weaning process. I would decide, he would cry, and I would surrender. I would begin and then stop again.

Within this rhythm, I knew that the only way to close this chapter would be for me to go cold turkey. So Jon and I packed our bags and took a road trip to Santa Barbara. Taking space while navigating a different form of attachment was necessary for Jupiter and me.

The L.A. sun shone brightly over the bustling city's horizon. On a typical spring day of 70 degrees and sunny, Jon and I packed our bags into our car. My emotions and resolve to finally wean ebbed between excitement, readiness, and dismay. Sure, I was elated to be done with nursing once and for all. However, I couldn't shake the all-consuming heaviness of the reality that this was it. This would be the last babe I would sustain with my body, who would find home within my breast while nuzzling close to my heart. Within our cozy cocoon, Jupiter and I sat on our twilled sofa, which we had found ourselves on many times before. He nursed for the last time as I counted his fingers and barefoot toes while I attempted to hold time captive. Cheek to chest, Jupiter extended his chocolate-colored fingers, lightly touching and framing my face, smiling wide-eyed and finding joy in his observation. He gazed at me as tears of both goodbye and "Mama, we made it" streamed down my face, finding their temporary dwelling within my collarbone. I repeatedly smelled the top of his head, offering a silent prayer that its scent would linger, although this moment would not.

I felt both joy and grief, proving that our feelings and emotions around growing are not monolithic but layered and complicated, shifting and changing. I cried tears of sadness and celebration. Though I knew it was time to reclaim my body as not just a mother but a human, I was still sad. We humans can feel both feelings at the same time. Grief and joy. Sad and happy. All of these emotions make up the evolution of our personhood. As I said my goodbyes, my heart broke.

What Are You Weaning? How Are You Soothing?

We all experience the weaning process whenever we let go or leave behind those things that no longer serve us. Weaning is the process that we all undergo when we close a chapter, simply because we feel within our bones that it has come to an end, much like an athlete who has pushed their body to the limit, attaining success and experiencing great triumph. When retiring, there is a season of letting go, and I am sure a time of weaning, from the training, two-a-days, and so much more.

Want to know if you are growing? Check in to see if there has been weaning. Weaning seasons are necessary if we are to abundantly grow. As our dreams expand and blossom, they require room to flourish. Our weaning holds our renewal. Weaning is the shedding of the old ways so that you can make space for the new.

At this point, I hope you've come to wean some of your survival tools that no longer serve you and instead are replacing them with healthier rituals.

Weaning was the end of our current nurturing relationship for Jupiter and me and the beginning of a new one. My identity had become intertwined within the foliage of either growing or nurturing a human. Like many, our identities become fixed against who we've shown ourselves to be versus who we are. I want you to know that it is possible to become depleted by what you may have found joy in many moons ago. Who we are and what we need within our ever-expanding identities shift. And that's okay. Our communities, family and friends, can support our weaning process, they may even see the need to do so before we do and lovingly nudge us along the way. I had a host of friends and sisters who saw the toll that daily breastfeeding had begun to take on my mental and emotional health. You may have friends who see it too. People who recognize the toil of continuing on and how free you could be and would be if you decided to just release. These friends gladly stepped in to support me as I let go. My sister friend watched the boys so I could step away for a few days to begin the weaning process. My colleagues in birth work congratulated me on a job well done and shared from their personal weaning experiences what I could expect now that I was on this new path.

We must give others the permission to grow, expand, and shed what no longer aligns, even if that means that we are a piece of that weaning. We are not who we were yesterday. And although weaning ain't easy, the result of remaining where growth is airless and stagnant is far more brutal.

Maybe you are in a relationship that has left you feeling depleted, and the more you progress along your self-intimacy journey, the more you realize that this relationship (platonic or romantic) no longer aligns with who you are and where you are growing. You may be in what used to be your dream career, and the longer you stay planted within the environment, the more you feel less like the person you are looking to become. This, too, calls for a weaning process, a breaking away from the title and our attachment to its importance. We outgrow our current groups and environments and hold on because they are all we know. Like my experience with weaning Jupiter, we produce every reason imaginable to continue on in attachment. "They are the only family I know." "Where else can I go?" "What if I fail?" We come up with reason after reason to remain tethered. However, sometimes we must wean to welcome.

Weaning can feel uneasy and awkward, as we fumble toward our footing. I ask, how are you soothing within the discomfort? Many of us soothe by distracting ourselves from the fear of the new and unknown path. We divert from the pang of separation. We seek perhaps the validation of others, affirming that we are on the "right path." Nature makes no announcement of change, nor does it notify the world when it grows. We live in an age of social media and instant gratification through validation, while nature has no desire or requirement to broadcast its movements. We could stand to learn a few things from nature. Nature simply is. An oak tree enters as a tiny seedling, growing in the dark beneath the earth. When expanding and weaning, notice how you soothe the discomfort within the change while buried beneath the soil. How do we soothe?

First, we recognize that weaning is expansion, gifting us space to welcome in more of what we now need, hope for, and desire. When weaning Jupiter, I had to find new ways of soothing him and myself. I was used to showing up in love and for my baby's needs this way. However, as I expanded, so did my need for respite and the reclamation of agency over my own body. And the same is true for you. How you found joy and comfort before may also shift within the new iteration of yourself. How you soothe may change. Second, we invite in ease and release unrealistic expectations of ourselves and others. Weaning may require that you pull back, go in, or discover some sludgy mesh of both. Timelines may be pushed as you find your way forward. Weaning is transient. This, too, shall pass.

Last, remember your story. Remind yourself of all the hard things you've already done to simply be here. How did weaning allow you to grow forward? How did you bloom, despite its initial discomfort? Who surrounded you? What resources did you call in? How can you parent yourself in this moment? Asking ourselves these questions is critical, as they can act as a salve and reminder that we have not only traveled here before but also thrived right here in this empty and perhaps undiscovered land.

COMMUNITY PARENTING

What comes to mind when you hear the term "community parenting"? Perhaps an image of 1960s commune life? Maybe your inclination is to skip ahead because birth and kids are not in your current or desired cards. Whatever your initial thought, I ask you to hang tight. Remember, when I use the term "parenting," I mean it in the most inclusive sense. We are all birthing/parenting something. We all need community to birth whatever we are trying to bring into the world. We are not supposed to go at this alone. Parenting ain't for punks, and it isn't for the faint of heart. Whether raising children or a dream, or simply adulting in this wild and crazy world, you need a community to thrive.

What is community parenting? It is a practice by which a child is looked after, cared for, and nurtured by various trusted adults in addition to parents. I'm sure you've likely heard the adage "It takes a village to raise a child"—community parenting is that village in action. But as adults, we can and should apply community parenting to ourselves as well. Who in your community helps to grow you?

When we look at African Indigenous villages, we see the communal model within the parenting relationship. A teacher and dear friend of mine, Aishat Hasati, shared with me this parental model during my pregnancy with Jupiter. She explained how within African tribes, parental responsibility is shared amongst the community. The mindset of simply "looking out" for and a village raising a child is the norm, not the exception to the rule. The burden of caring about and for your child and vice versa is the village's collective calling.

Simply put, when I see your child, I see my own. When you see my child, you respond as if they are yours. Within this communal rhythm, nothing is missing or lacking. I would also imagine that because there are so many loving arms and hearts toward the family, the space for impostor syndrome arising is minimal, as the support is present. Whatever I don't know, my sister or brother knows and vice versa. There is no gap left unfilled within this intentional bond.

The same community model is not only valid for raising children, it also applies to birthing our visions and dreams. Humans are communal beings, and much like our plant friends, we thrive best when we are operating within communities. Allow your village to come alongside your reparenting journey, calling on those who have been where you are. The beauty of community parenting is that we don't have to have all the answers, as the answers are found alongside and in connection and openness with one another.

What does creating this village look like in adulthood, and how do we find it? I can tell you that it's located in our collective circles, friends that become family, and upon the sofas of therapists and other healing modalities that nurture our souls. If I were to comprise a checklist of sorts, at the top, the prerequisite is that these people support us in our self-discovery and want to see us achieve our highest good and become our most whole selves. I like to think of those who community parent alongside us as co-laborers, co-waterers, and, dare I say, participants in our birth work or our doulas. These people come alongside us, whether we are birthing an objective or encountering a rebirth of ourselves. Like doulas, they hold our hand as we labor through the complex parts of life and celebrate when we accomplish what we weren't sure was possible. This circle can also be found in moments of disappointment and heavy loss, reminding us after the first, second, and even third attempts that birthing our wildest dreams is still possible for us.

How do we create this community of parenting? These relationships work best when they form organically and remain unforced yet intentional. They also work best when they are rooted in reciprocity and there is an equal energy exchange. And please note, when I say equal, I don't mean the exchange will look identical. Because we all come with our unique ways of holding space, supporting, and showing up. However, we should all feel respected and valued within this collaborative relationship. Much like roses and garlic, we each nourish and protect each other from a cold and careless world.

How do we open ourselves up to community parenting? We make ourselves available for support even when we want to isolate. You may be used to solving problems alone. Community parenting says you don't have to.

· · · · · · · · · ·

In my early years of parenthood, I suffered from significant impostor syndrome and felt like a fraud. I would love to say that impostor syndrome was new for me. However, it wasn't. I carried it long before becoming a parent, and I continued to bring it into my career opportunities and overall work.

I'll never forget making the conscious decision to channel my inner Beyoncé and quit my job. I was working in the fashion industry, supplying textiles to local brands. I had recently given birth to my second son, Jedi, and was struggling with the balance of meetings and client demands, all while carrying a babe on my back. En route to and from work errands, I'd pull over in my car every five minutes to nurse my baby in the backseat. Baby Jedi hated riding in the car and would scream bloody murder every time we went for a ride. I was worn down and experienced weekly panic attacks. I also felt a deep calling for a career shift and in my overall purpose. I began hosting small gatherings, writing and sharing my experience with miscarriage, creating new community and indulging in the stories of others. It was the beginning stages of what would become Moms in Color, a collective created to celebrate diversity and intersectional motherhood.

Somewhere between creating these new pathways for connection and balancing the next wave of anxiety, I knew it was time to pivot. This old way was no longer the path forward for me. I could feel it. So much so that my body was telling me through sensation after sensation. Been there? I felt a pull, a tug toward my future and the ease I so desperately wanted to experience in my life and work. It was time to move forward. But how? This is where community parenting comes into play. Much like a person who is pregnant, I began to do the following:

- I shared the big news! I told trusted friends that I wanted to create a space for people to share life's beautiful and complex parts. I was still determining what it would entail and how to accomplish it. However, I knew that what I didn't have knowledge of, someone within my village surely would.

- With my trusted community, I shared where I was in my goal's pregnancy, my fears, and the parts that felt like dead ends and insecurities.

- I didn't have everything I needed to move forward with this dream. However, gathering a team of people or community parents would prove beneficial. We can be completely open with these people, creating clear signposts to how they can support us according to their role.

Five People You Need in Community Parenting While Birthing and Raising Your Dream:

1. The Teacher. This can be someone who knows more than you about what you want to achieve and can point you in the right direction when you are stuck. Again, this modality of care ensures that we don't have to have all the answers.

2. The Accountant (not money-related). Someone who will hold you accountable for what you say you will do. These are the folk who will gently remind us when we get off course, helping to guide us back. And when we intentionally shift, they are the ones who will show us grace in the new path forward while still holding us to it.

3. The Hole Puncher. This person's job is to poke holes. To ask the question, "Have you considered _____?"

Please note that this person should be someone you trust, as their job is to offer productive critiques. Their whole purpose in support is to honestly want the best for you and from you.

4. The Nurturer. These people are our life doulas. They coach and help us navigate hard moments that feel weighty while birthing. They are here to comfort us while reminding us that we've made it through tough things before and survived many of our hardest days. These nurturers come in handy when on our path we hit a snag, a dead end, or what some may call a fail, a.k.a. a temporary detour.

5. The Healthy Distractor. I know. When you hear the word "distraction," you are likely wondering how this can be a good thing. To that, I offer because sometimes not only do we need a break (which our nurturer can give), but we need to step away and do something that has nothing to do with anything except simply stepping away. Sometimes we need to temporarily distract ourselves from goals and timelines and just be, go for a walk without our cellphone and no brainstorming, just a conversation about the sky and a meme about a cute puppy.

REPARENTING AND OUR ENVIRONMENT

As I mentioned, I have nearly fifty plants. One summer, I was trying to find the right home for one of my many ferns. She moved around the house until I figured a place in the sun with her fellow ferns would work best. She, too, needed her (fern) friends in order to grow and thrive within the space. What we are surrounded by, our proximity to the growth and nurturing needed, plays a part in our thriving. When you purchase a new plant, it is recommended that the plant not be repotted until it has time to acclimate to its new environment. Before moving into its new pot home, it must first settle into its new surroundings. The same is true for us humans. Our soil environment is everything. Being intentional within our movements is vital to our growth, as our surroundings can significantly affect our thriving.

When you are nurturing your vision, what does your environment or community tell you? Does it encourage the development of your dream? Are you moving too fast, changing your space unintentionally, because that's what the clock says? Managing our surrounding ecosystems is how we thrive. As the Beatles said, we get by—and thrive—with a little help from our friends.

1. Name immediate and actionable ways that you can begin reparenting yourself. What are you seeking? What are your needs? Identify ways you can provide emotional self-provision.
2. Right here. Right now. How can you show up for yourself in radical tenderness?
3. What are you weaning? How are you soothing?
4. Finish this sentence: Reparenting myself looks like _____.
5. Locate your village. Who are your five people?

PART TWO

···

Matters of the Mind

GLORIA, THE SNAKE PLANT

Snake plants are resilient, their thriving does not require much, but what they do need is consistency. Snake plants know how to be their own place of safety.

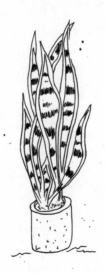

CHAPTER SIX

Finding Safety Post-Trauma

I met a woman at a retreat who asked a very exact yet almost unanswerable question, after hearing about my work. At least not an answer that I could quickly summarize in a few sentences and quotes. She shared how her childhood home was a strange land filled with abuse, addiction, and emotional neglect. Her mother was an addict and would oftentimes put her in harm's way as a child, along with herself. She shared how she would find her mom passed out on the sofa from drug usage or drinking. There were no bedtime stories and forehead kisses before gently turning off her Rainbow Brite lamp meticulously placed on top of her bedside table. As a child, she was designated somewhat as her mother's caretaker. She would witness and encounter traumatic experiences where she too had to be ten times smarter than her adult, often using her childlike survival skills and wit to prevent danger, tragic endings, and even house fires. She shared that her father, whom she would later lose in adulthood, was her only source of safety within her home. Within the disarray and madness of addiction and pain, he was her safe space.

And at this retreat, filled with trees and open sky, the woman asked me the question that I couldn't fully answer in one sitting. She asked, how did I find my way back? How did I find my way to feelings of safety past the trauma? Past the corridors of no return after seeing what you can never unsee and the fear that you can never quite untaste? I assured her that it wasn't one singular experience but instead a symphony of a million moments working together to carry and build me back safely, post-trauma.

Some of us have never known what it feels like to experience this kind of safety. This moment of "after" or even during the storm. I can tell you that this feeling of security afterward feels like home. A home that, although we may have never crossed its doorstep before, we all know exists and is there waiting for us to discover. Safety is there for us to feel its warmth, welcoming us in after a long day of just living. Some of us have never felt the embrace of its walls and protection of its fortresses. I was one of those people. I dedicate this chapter to the woman who asked me this question.

We, the Undone

Healing is not a destination.
It is a journey.

Before we move forward, I want you to know that this work is not a set destination but a continuous journey. We are all what I like to call "the undone." We are all unfinished and unfixed artistry. Many people feel that regaining our mental health post-trauma, or in spite of it, is perhaps a one-stop. We look for quick fixes and elixirs to numb our feelings, feelings that we must experience to heal. We adorn ourselves with crystals and all sorts of external remedies, forgetting that we are the real magic. Then we become thrown off by triggers and begin to assume that we are "doing it wrong" when that couldn't be further from the case. Do you recognize your triggers? Well, that's a step in the right direction. Embracing this undone state allows endless learning opportunities and cultivates empathy toward yourself and others. Remember, undone means that there is still more to learn and embody. When one is finished, there is nothing left.

We often hear the phrase "Time heals all wounds." I don't believe that to be true. I think that often we trade in time for neglect, hoping that somehow the clock will heal our hearts, and often it does not. In fact, as with any wound, if left untreated, it can produce additional problems and infection. Our hearts and minds are no different. Time does not heal all wounds. Doing the work heals all wounds.

Suppose you are having a hard time beginning, or perhaps even wanting, to embark on this journey. You are not lazy, complacent, or any of the other terms that folks like to throw around when people find themselves stuck. Healing trauma and practicing true resilience is hard, backbreaking work. I get it. However, if there's one thing I can offer you, doing the work and digging through what no longer aids our growth is well worth it. One of my favorite quotes is Mobb Deep's "There's a war going on outside no man is safe from." Which sums up trauma. We all experience some form of war, whether externally or internally. The healing looks different for all. However, it is our responsibility to pursue it.

Where does it hurt?
Open the wound and let the sunlight in.

THE RESILIENCE OF FLOWERS AND US

Succulents are mad resilient. I know, what a way to begin.

When I think of the woman who asked me about mending post-trauma, I am reminded of my snake plant, Gloria. I purchased Gloria on the corner in a random neighborhood of Los Angeles. When I bought her, her stalks were long and lean, resembling spears that reached the heavens. I traveled outside of town to pick her up from an online ad. Why? I don't know, one would think that going to the plant and garden store down the street would have been enough. It was not. I brought her home, placing her first on the floor, then near a window, and finally on a stool adjacent to my fiddle fig, Tina. Gloria's soil was different from that of my other plants. It was rocky, filled with pebbles and loose dirt, instead of the smooth, rich planting soil where some of my plants made their home. Gloria was a bit of a badass. She was sharp and jagged, and if you made a wrong move while kneeling to water her fellow plants, she could poke you in the eye. The stone-filled dirt was her home. Gloria was absolutely rock-and-roll incarnate, if that is even possible for plants. If she were a person, she would be the kid in school who was defiant, not just because, but because it was their right to push, shove, and discover their way to the daylight.

Now, I will say for Gloria to have been so bold, she somehow always seemed to find herself as the lucky recipient of her dirt being pulled from underneath her, courtesy of my youngest child Jupiter's excavating. I would sweep the misplaced earth from the floor, placing it back into Gloria's pot. I would apologize to her, begging her forgiveness and assuring her that my three-year-old Jupiter knew not what he had done. Then the occasional book from the bookshelf would fall on her leaves, bending them. I was also guilty of forgetting to water her. However, if anyone knows about the many perks of succulents, they are desert plants and don't require a lot of watering or care. They have adapted to their surroundings of needing less maintenance and attention. I would forget to do and provide for Gloria. Leaf by leaf would begin to droop, slowly dying as I not only neglected her, but as the boys flung toys at her. At one point, her leaves lay flat against her pot and were no longer upright. She begged me to water her, place her back into the sun, or at least place her in a spot where she was no longer subject to danger and trauma.

I had seen this happen with a few of my plants. They would experience the traumatic event of scarcity, or an object being hurled full speed at them, and they would indeed seem as though they'd die from the brunt of their exposure. Sometimes I'd sit the plant outside for a bit before making the unfortunate decision to finally dump its remains into either the garbage or the front yard. However, I didn't want to throw Gloria away, even though I was sure that trauma had rendered this plant done. There were no longer stems bursting through the soil. No leaves were reaching toward the light, only dirt. I sat Gloria on my porch and walked away, forgetting about her. I was confident that I ultimately killed this plant, as there were no signs of life, only the rubble of earth.

A few weeks later, I noticed something happening. Leaves had started to peek through the dirt. And it wasn't just one or two leaves. Multiple leaves began sprouting through as if they had been there all along. This plant was not dead and most certainly was not done. This plant was resilient. It had done exactly what plants are supposed to do. It made its way to the light and grew. It thrived.

The thing that I love most about plants is their resilience.

There was a study published by the journal *New Phytologist* that took note of the resilience of flowers. Like us, many of them experience significant trauma, causing their stems to bend and petals to fall. Somehow these same flowers find the will to not only live but bend themselves back to where they once were, reorienting themselves. This recalibration is fundamental with flowers, because if they don't bend themselves back, then their chance of pollination is slim. No pollination equals no reflowering of their community. Plants were dispositioned to survive and thrive no matter what, implementing their resilience because of survival. We are no different. Like all living things, we humans possess this same resilience.

RESILIENCE, THE R-WORD

Truthfully, I become a little leery even mentioning the word "resilience." When I hear it so often and so casually placed upon the backs of those who have had to be strong and, dare I say it, resilient, throughout their lives and within their bodies, I cringe at the thought of using it. I know that many people who have had to be resilient shouldn't have to be. We unintentionally make excuses for abusive behaviors and enduring such, all in the name of resilience. We also subscribe to unhealthy environments and toxic cultures in the name of resilience. So, I want to first and foremost state for the record my personal belief when it comes to the R-word, our friend, and I believe superpower, resilience.

Resilience is not about how much we can grin and bear the tough things that come at us. I don't believe nor subscribe to simply celebrating how much you can take or endure without dying, slowly deteriorating from the weight of it all. I believe that resilience is about recognizing the power we all have within us, like the purple lilies or the hardy succulent, holding it between our hands. Resilience is the audacity to grow regardless of what we have encountered. It is not about how stoically we can take hit after hit, but instead the nerve by which we take back our power, straightening our stems and growing. It is the gumption to continue cultivating safety within ourselves.

You hold the resilience of flowers.
You, too, possess the audacity to grow.

Your environment determines your capacity for blooming.
Check your soil.
Check your potting.
Check your space.

MATTERS OF THE MIND

A large part of my decision to seek therapy after Jon's infidelity was to indeed check the soil of my mind, as my anxiety had moved on to what felt like full-on depression. And I have to say, depression felt different. It felt like a load I had never carried before, despite what I had previously seen or witnessed. My arms were heavy. Depression felt scary and unfamiliar. Anxiety, I knew what that was. It felt like the bear chasing me through the alley or in my home. But depression felt like a whole slew of zoo animals had finally caught up with me, sitting on my chest, and suffocating whatever joy or light there was left in the world.

Anxiety felt brash. It would flood my system as it crashed

against me like loud, boisterous cymbals in a marching band. Anxiety, although familiar, would make its announcement every time it entered the room. "Here we are again," it said as it sounded its tuba, marching across the living room floor.

For me, depression was more subtle and sneaky. It would begin with a thought, a paralyzing "what-if" that would freeze me in my tracks and lock me within the room of fear. Depression can feel insular and opaque. Thoughts become foggy as you sink into its remote nature. Perhaps your limbs and body feel heavy. I've found that for some who lack a name for the initial churning feeling of anxiety and the acknowledgment of trauma experienced, the despair of it all sets in, swallowing one whole while pushing further and further into depression. For me, when anxiety pivoted into depression, I had a more challenging time calling this by name. Perhaps it was the stigma surrounding it. Many people who navigate anxiety find themselves dealing with depression at some point. The therapy world calls anxiety depression's close relative. When the fear is unchecked and unhealed, it eventually becomes despair. Which then can spiral to depression, and that's where I was then.

I had seen up close and personal how depression could present from a parent. In between my father's ever-changing moods, he would sink into moments of deep depression. And although his version of depression didn't resemble covers pulled over his head, his, like many men's, looked and felt like anger, violence, and irritability, all while pushing us away. It looked like tears and the contemplation of no longer being here. And this heaviness toward life and all-consuming rage muddied my scope a bit of what depression could also mean for you and me and that it shows itself in many forms. When you think of depression, what are some of the passenger thoughts that come to mind?

Because of my experience, the passenger thought I carried was that depression was for the mentally unstable and the unwell. It was for the unproductive and inconsolable. I was working and writing, parenting and managing. My life and actions didn't resemble the passenger thoughts I'd picked up around depression. Yet there I was, overperforming, overachieving, and so very depressed.

I was diagnosed with generalized anxiety at the age of thirty-nine. After years of feeling the continual motor of my brain running and feeling exhausted from the recurring panic attacks, I finally decided to talk with a psychiatrist. Funny enough, having a name put to what I had attempted to pray away, jog away, and combat with happy thoughts was a wave of relief. Being able to call it by its name felt liberating instead of the nonstop spiral of what I experienced. Dear reader, when you know your wounds by name, you begin to understand them intimately and their origins. And then maybe, just maybe, you can become friends with them. I believe one of the greatest labors in our lives is our mental well-being, which requires acknowledging and understanding the trauma we have experienced.

As we have talked about, from childhood to adulthood, we experience moments that either wound or help develop us, and as we mature somewhere along the way, we must find a place where we can revisit what happened to us, hold compassion for ourselves as we experienced it, and then from that place live alongside it, as we cannot alter the past. I want this time together to be spent on you coming to terms with what's hindering your thriving regarding your own mental health. Is it the stigmas and passenger thoughts we discussed in the preceding chapter? Maybe it's the fear of being labeled as depressed, a victim, or the proud recipient of an anxiety disorder diagnosis.

Our Mental Health: the Wellspring

Our mental health includes our emotional, psychological, and social well-being. Our mental health is the wellspring from which all things flow, affecting all we touch. How we prioritize our mental health may look different for everyone, but it starts with an awareness that we are worthy of a life that exists beyond survival and that we all need support to realize it fully. Truthfully, the ways we implement that support are up to our choosing. However, I believe it begins with us all asking the simple question "What is the life I want to live?" And for clarification, I'm not referring to the monetary or tangible items we wish to possess. I am simply asking the elementary question. What is the life you wish to live, not merely despite trauma, but in response to it? A life of peace? Rebellious thriving? Adventure and bravery?

I knew it was time to attend to my mental health when I finally felt overrun, unable to find myself within the overgrown ivy of anxiety and depression. The light that grew despite the darkness began to dim. My thoughts felt foggy. I assumed this was because of children and exhaustion. Until I saw those around me who seemed to live a life not so filled with anxiety. They seemed lighter. Sure, these people, friends and associates, had also experienced grief, loss, their version of despair, and everything we humans experience. Yet somehow they seemed to know how to feel the heaviness of all the parts and still make peace with it. I knew that if I didn't take notice of my mental health, I could risk being devoured by it. I wasn't okay. Adult trauma on top of childhood trauma had me questioning what I was doing here. This life of constant triggers and gritted teeth, as I tried to ignore the origin of harm, couldn't be all there was to life. I wasn't sleeping well but had also chalked it up to the fact that I had kids, as opposed to the remnants of the many nights of me as a child being woken out of my sleep by midnight fights and their memory stored deep.

As I started visualizing myself on the other side of trauma, it wasn't a depiction of someone without past trauma, nor was it of someone who had forgotten it. I simply saw myself as someone who desired to no longer see life through its darkened and trauma-filled lens. Maybe not at first glance, but hopefully eventually.

I am not referring to mental illness through chemical imbalance, such as bipolar disorder, schizophrenia, or personality disorders. These are conditions outside my experience, and I don't feel comfortable draping a one-size-fits-all blanket across them. I will also say that this is not about curing anything or anyone. I am simply addressing the residual effects of how we adapt to survive post-trauma. I am sharing my realizations so that you can thrive while navigating your own mental health.

Maybe for you, it isn't anxiety or depression. Instead, it's a constant worry, a never-ending churning that never goes away. Again, you are worthy of a life not rooted in simply making it through. Your life is yours to enjoy.

IDENTIFY THE TRIGGERS

To start locating our safety and taking back our plantlike resilient power, we must first know our triggers. I like to imagine triggers as trees. Tall and broad, their leaves and branches cascading the atmosphere. Like trees, triggers are everywhere. And quite frankly, home, safety, and those we love are not exempt from possibly triggering us. The foliage from our triggers touch each other, often getting in the way, blinding us from our present home, past our transient triggers. It is not enough to simply know our triggers but to be familiar with them and our worthiness in choosing, embodying, and allowing the present to greet us. When we are familiar with our triggers and encounter them within safe spaces, we can properly place them as perhaps faultless, communicate them, and see them for what they are—trees within the broader (and still safe) forest. Becoming familiar with our triggers prevents those same triggers from robbing us of our present life and current happiness.

Knowing our triggers allows us to be kind to ourselves and encourages us to live in awareness of others. By simply acknowledging our triggers, we can begin to be mindful that we all have an internal dialogue constantly taking place, telling us that we are not good enough or worthy enough. These triggers remind us that we all have suitcases that we are continually unpacking, folding the contents of, and politely putting away for no one to see.

I know. After you have walked along this healing journey, I wish I could say that triggers vanish into the abyss. However, we all know that that is not true. Triggers persist, primarily because of trauma. We're in traffic, and a nearby driver flips us off. We are then triggered by the times we've felt dismissed or cast away. Our co-worker got the position we wanted at the job. We are then activated by times in our childhood when we felt overlooked and rejected. You lost your keys, and you are reminded of all the times you have encountered loss. Triggers are present and serve as a reminder of all the places by which healing is needed.

As a birth and postpartum doula, I have witnessed clients' triggers quite frequently. Clients who had experienced a childhood riddled with violence and abuse, grasping for the one thing we have no power over during childbirth: control. Clients who had encountered the aches of grief now experience the same in labor as they'd cry out for those lost. One thing about birth and postpartum that was reasonably predictable was that triggers were inevitable. So much so that during my time with the expectant parents, I would get to know them intimately. Before touching their feet or hands to provide acupressure, I would ask them if I had their consent. Was it okay for me to rub their back while supporting possible discomfort? I knew that for those who had experienced sexual abuse and/or assault, the simple act of touch without consent (even during birth support) could be triggering, signaling to my client's nervous system that they were in danger again.

Birth of any kind calls for a specific vulnerability that many are not aware of until they are in it. And if there's one thing that also springs forth triggers, it's vulnerability, the unknown, and the uncontrollable. (All of which sum up the birthing experience.) Trying something new? Be prepared that triggers will remind you of all the times you've attempted and failed.

Being a birth guide left me entrenched in triggers of my own. After my second miscarriage, I ventured back in the world to support a postpartum parent while I, too, was postpartum. But this time without a baby to show for it. I didn't mention to my client that I had just suffered a miscarriage a week earlier, as I tried not to muddy my work life with the personal. So much so that as part of a ritual, I would enter a client's home and immediately wash my hands. Of course, I'd do this for health reasons whenever interacting with a newborn. But I would also do this as a ritual to wash away everything on my hands and heart as I entered my client's home. I was there to support them. And for that moment, I needed to be free of anything that didn't do just that.

I remember holding my client's little one as the parents would nourish themselves, gobbling down the food I had prepared as if it had been days since they had eaten in peace. More than likely it had. I cradled their baby's head within the crook of my arm as they clasped their tiny hand around my index finger. Their belly pressed against my now empty womb. Cue trigger. While I was in this beautiful moment of supporting this family (newborns are seriously one of the best perks of this work), I was reminded of how I'd looked forward to holding my own baby. This moment of wonder triggered the remembrance of loss and what was supposed to be. Triggers are profound in this way. They are birthed both in joyful moments and in longing. And in a deep wish that things were just, quite simply, different.

And while I could tell you step-by-step what I did, the first and most crucial part was allowance. I allowed myself to feel the achy part and longing. Triggers can serve as a beautiful reminder that healing is still needed in a specific area of our lives. And where healing is requested, gentleness is required. When we acknowledge that we have hurt and that there is an area seeking repair, we will in turn begin to show kindness to ourselves in that specific area that is being activated or triggered.

So what do we do when history shows up to dance with our current reality? Remember that triggers serve a purpose. I remember reading from a dear friend via social media regarding insecurities: "Insecurities are not there to mock you. They are here to show you where you need healing." I would say the same is true of triggers. Though uncomfortable, perhaps triggers are not all bad. Perhaps triggers are there to protect, to remind, and to heal.

You are safe, even though you feel out of control. I can often feel the fear reverberating off my clients as they fight through the surrender that the birthing experience demands. Stroking their hair, I remind them, "You are safe. You are safe. You are safe. Listen, we've all been there. Things go left, and immediately we feel pummeled in the uncertainty. I want you to know that you can feel safe within the unknown." Eventually, I can feel the tension leave my client's body as they surrender.

Remember your agency. Our choice is the first thing to go when experiencing trauma. It vanishes along with our agency. I found that a considerable part of my thriving was reclaiming my intuitive sense of choice. There were so many times during the trauma of my younger years that left me stranded without choice. Anxiety would rise, and the first thing I would feel leave my presence was my sense of choice. I'm sure you feel it too. Remembering that I have a sense of agency is a powerful tool in my thriving toolkit. I thrive during triggers by reminding myself that I have choice in my corner, agency, and reserve the right to choose. I may not like the specific options presented, but I can still choose, and so can you. Ask yourself what your choices are at this moment, and see what the door opens up to reveal.

Your sense of agency is the one thing this life cannot loot. People are going to be people, and life will live its best. There are more factors outside your control than within it. Choice not only influences how we move through this world, but if we are unaware of its existence, it can keep us prisoner to past traumas, condemning us to relive them repeatedly. I want you to know that what you genuinely possess in this world is your power of intention and how you wish to proceed from the initial trauma, disappointment, and distress. You may ask, "How does my sense of agency connect with my mental health?" Reclaiming your agency is like gathering all the broken pieces within your hands, touching them, and fully knowing that the brokenness of the fragments no longer mirrors who you are. We can choose from a place of now. Choice is how you reclaim your time, being, and belonging.

Connection and Co-Regulation. Triggers can feel isolating. You may think that no one could possibly understand what you are feeling. Maybe they can't. However, I want you to know that you are not alone, even in your triggers. Dr. Mona Delahooke says, "Co-regulation is the dance between two nervous systems, each mirroring the other's movements and emotions, creating a harmonious rhythm of attunement and connection." Amazingly, allowing those around us into our triggers can create calm within our dysregulated nervous system. Co-regulation is a powerful tool that enables individuals to work together with the intent to regulate their current trauma responses, emotions, and dysregulated nervous system. It is demonstrated through physical and emotional cues, feedback, and mutual responses, signaling that safety is present while offering connection instead of isolation. Humans are not meant to function in isolation. Co-regulation affirms this, as it supports us as we labor through challenging moments together.

An example of co-regulation: Two friends may be respectively triggered, but instead of responding via trauma response, empathy and validation of each other's perspective are offered. This offering of listening and empathy calms both people's nervous systems. In short, my self-regulation provides a safe space for your nervous system and vice versa.

Please note that co-regulation should not be confused with co-dependence. Here is the difference between the two: Co-regulation is exhibited when all individuals work *together* to regulate their emotions and nervous systems. In contrast, in co-dependence, an individual leans solely on the other for this support. There is no mutual exchange. Co-dependency and thriving are like oil and water. They don't mix.

Show gratitude. After all, our triggers are simply doing their job. Many years ago, water found its way to my laptop. I watched as my computer powered down slowly from the waterlogged keys. I want to say that I reacted coolly, calmly, and collectedly. I did not. Feelings of not only frustration but regret and sadness began to surface. I began to cry, not just because of the possibility of having to purchase a new laptop, but because this was yet again something that I might lose. This trigger was a reminder that I have experienced loss on a far deeper level than a possibly waterlogged laptop, and that I can feel deeply in this area and connect with others who have gone through this shared experience because of this loss. Triggers allow us to be kind to ourselves and encourage us to live in awareness of others. By simply acknowledging our triggers, we can begin to be mindful that we all have an internal dialogue constantly taking place, telling us that we are not good enough or worthy enough and that "this is why we can't have nice things."

Here's a quick list to process through:

1. Identify your passenger thoughts around mental health. Do these passenger thoughts currently support your mental health?
2. What does life look like when you visualize yourself on the other side of trauma?
3. Identify your triggers. How do you usually move through them?
4. Recognize where co-regulation can be implemented as a supportive tool.

CHAPTER SEVEN

Replacing Surviving Tools
with Thriving Tools

Recognizing our survival tools is key to moving forward in our mental health journey. Survival tools are often what we use to mitigate triggers and attempt to keep ourselves safe. Survival tools are directly connected to our initial wound; they are all the mechanisms we've gathered to survive this life, unlike our thriving tools, which demand more, desiring to thrive and relish on this side of paradise, not merely survive it.

As you'll recall, on my psychedelic trip, I saw the lifeless statue-like figure that I grasped as if my life depended on it. I realized that this replica of myself was a tool I had picked up for my survival. As a child, I needed this tool, this statue, to navigate and outlast the dangers around me. When we notice how we survive, we can better understand where and why we are the way we are. The opposite is also true. When we do not recognize our survival tools, the pattern of surviving and spiraling continues.

It will be helpful to spend some time recognizing some of the most common survivor tools I've witnessed. If we pass by your street while doing so, sit with this tool and what you'd like to replace it with.

SURVIVAL TOOLS FOR PERCEIVED SAFETY

Fear of being seen. Often, our tools for survival are centered on an immediate, almost innate response and relief of triggers and the past trauma experienced. So, for example, when I would feel a threat of danger making its appearance, I would resort to what I knew.

Protect and hide all the knives. Think through and rule out every possible chance of trouble, which would then send me into a tailspin of the additional potential danger of which to be aware. I would build my trusted fortress around me, shielding me from all possible harm. I've observed that the threat of danger looks different post-trauma. The risk is no longer simply resolved to physical or emotional harm, but includes the simple act of being seen. You may say, "Well, everyone wants to be seen." And yes, for the most part, you are correct. However, for those who have experienced the unthinkable such as the trauma of violence, being seen is not so painless, nor does it necessarily feel safe. To allow others to see us, we must be vulnerable, which after experiencing what we've experienced, we vowed never to leave ourselves open to again. Vulnerability requires that we share our thoughts and how we feel, and to do such a thing means we must offer what we have held on to for dear life. If no one knows how we feel, that is not only one more thing that helps keep ourself safe but one less thing that perhaps those who possess the capability of harming us have. I want you to know that building castle-like fortresses and moats for those who love us to cross is a trauma response. Allowing our past to act as guards keeping us safe within our tower, all in the name of not being fully seen, is also a trauma response. However, I want you to know that the moment we decide to be fully seen, that is the moment we allow support, understanding, and a witness to our beautiful humanity.

Avoidance of being seen looks like this:

1. Emotional avoidance. When conversation calls for you to be emotionally transparent, you deflect.
2. Avoidance of hard conversations. You would rather sever a relationship than be vulnerable.
3. Avoidant eye contact. We've heard it said before. Eyes are windows to the soul. When we peer into each other's eyes and allow others to see into ours, it grants permission to be seen. Shifting our eyes away cuts off communication that courses beyond our perhaps fearfully edited words.

Self-sabotage. Anaïs Nin said, "We don't see things as they are. We see them as we are." This idea is a perfect example of trauma response and its survival tools instead of the thriving means we can acquire. Often, when we have experienced substantial trauma, we build up a resistance to good things happening. We will sabotage, deflect, even resist as if what is happening for us is not ours to possess. I've been there. As mentioned, a considerable part of this work that I embarked upon was because I wanted to begin claiming the things finding their way to me as my own. Often, our trauma creates blocks and hurdles for us to accept the gift of good. Because of our experiences, we feel unworthy of it. We agonize and imagine the worst-case scenario because trauma has groomed us to believe that nothing ever works out, not for people like you and me. This bracing ourselves is a survival tool adapted because of trauma. If we brace ourselves for impact, the fall feels lighter and won't kill us.

Self-sabotage is a common feature of many who have encountered the trauma of abandonment, violence, early childhood attachment wounds and neglect, and the chronic disappointment that raises its head after that. We wear it like a cloak, draped across our back, but often have no recognition that it lives here within our beliefs and practices. Self-sabotage creates skipped opportunities, as we allow them to stay orphaned and unclaimed at the doorway. Self-sabotage slams the door shut before it has a chance to open. Self-sabotage, although seldom identified, is a coping method presented to deal with the residue of our trauma. I describe it as the blanket we snuggle under to make us feel less in danger and a little less afraid.

Not all survival tools resemble a bottle to our lips or a needle to our arm. Your means of surviving can also look like a wash and repeat of past trauma, reintroducing it repeatedly. However, this method of coping is just as destructive to ourself and our future.

Although they may be unrecognizable, I believe the effects of self-sabotage feel all too familiar. Because of trauma, we create the reality we see ourselves deserving of and accustomed to. Familiarity and its pull are full-bodied. If you are accustomed to chaos, self-sabotage looks like not only looking for it but creating it and perhaps unknowingly pulling the trigger on self-inflicted trauma to cope with the new normal of stability.

And listen, I understand. When we are triggered and in a state of flight or fight, what we cozy up to is often not what we would choose if we were actively aware of how it perpetuates further harm, nor would it be our first option. However, that awareness is precisely the key. Perhaps circumstances beyond your control took the power of intention—how you soothed created origins all in the name of survival and out of fear. You now get to choose how you fare in the distresses of life and how you mend. And when we can do this, we become closer to our true selves. Self-sabotage prevents us from fully becoming who we were always meant to be, as it is entrenched in fear. Ask yourself, who would you be without fear? What would you do? Self-sabotage prevents us from hearing the answer.

Examples of Self-Sabotage

1. Quitting. I will leave _____ before it has time to leave me. Abandonment is often the cause of this survival tool (but, of course, not limited to). Being abandoned is traumatic, often leaving recipients questioning their worth and worthiness of connection and meaningful relationship. "Why would anything good happen for me?" is a recurrent passenger thought.

2. Avoidance of trying. Those who adopt self-sabotage as a survival tool often possess the buried belief that good things only happen to others. Why try? After all, it's not going to happen. The root of this response is often fear of disappointment. The chance of rejection or a supposed negative result outweighs the option of not only trying, but that good could also be an outcome.

3. I will hurt you before you hurt me. We've all heard the expression "Hurt people hurt people." And it is so very true. People who exhibit hurtful behavior are often victims of harm themselves. Your interpersonal relationships are limited. Your survival tool is to hurt as a means of defense, to be the one who offers the final blow before you are knocked off your feet onto the ground. You may also avoid healthy intimate relationships.

4. You create self-inflicted trauma, willfully walking into known harm.

BUILDING WALLS

During therapy, I shared how childhood had left me petrified of everything and everyone around me and how it seemed to be a wall between the world and me, a wall that I had erected to keep me safe from it and the foes who inhabited it. I shared with my therapist how my stepfather, birth sister, stepsisters, and step-brother had a family text thread. They would text back and forth, commenting on their day and checking in. I also shared how I wouldn't respond. I was not too fond of text threads and re-quested that my family members no longer include me on the family thread. I chalked this request up to what seemed to be an insignificant ask and my boundaries. Translation: I don't like text threads, please respect my boundaries—the end. Case closed. However, this desire to distance myself from family was not cre-ating boundaries or a safe space, but instead altogether avoid-ance, an emotional defense mechanism that many folks who have encountered trauma put in place to keep them safe from the environment around them.

As a child, the feelings I experienced around my new siblings were simple. I felt alone. By the time my mom and stepdad in-troduced them into my life, I had already seen so much. The homelessness of my emotions and the aftershocks from the mo-lestation furthered the void between my siblings and me. In my head, they were able to play freely. Free from carrying the bur-den of secret and past pain. They didn't seem to have to work through the deficit of trauma. I had to pretend while playing pretend. From what I knew, they did not. And now, as an adult, every time my phone would ding, I would be reminded of this game of hiding the truth and seeking normalcy. I would build a wall. I and all of my broken trauma were on the outside. My siblings were inside, as they were not safe, as no one was safe. I resented them for their privilege to be kids, not seeming to carry the weight of what I had taken on so young. And while I didn't wish what I experienced as a child on my worst enemy, I wanted permission not to feel alone in my silence.

ANXIETY AS A MEANS OF SURVIVAL

The statue that I witnessed on my psychedelic trip was neither good nor bad. It was nothing and none of the labels that I had spoken over it for so very long. The anxiety was a survival tool adapted that now lay lifeless, almost like an erected mausoleum holding the dead. And what I gleaned from witnessing it was that my anxiety, too, was not bad. It was simply a solution, a call-and-response to the trauma experienced. It was there to keep me safe for as long as I needed it, releasing it when I did not. Knowing that these things were my brain's way of keeping me safe allowed me to view anxiety as not something to fix but something to hold with empathy and gratitude. I also recognized the immense amount of shame that I carried around my struggle with the internal dialogue in my head. It was as if no one must know my dirty little secret, so I buried it beneath the earth where all the dirty things go.

Like the replica of myself that I witnessed, I want you to know that your response to trauma is not who you are but merely an adaptogen to the trauma experienced. Nothing is wrong with *you*. These means of adaptation and survival kept you here, which is worth celebrating. As I stared at the replica of myself, I saw that while it looked exactly like me, it was not me. And to that I offer you the same: Your response to trauma is not who you are. You are not your anxiety. Your depression. Your worry. Despite all of the trauma you experienced, you were able to find your way to the light and survive. Now let's get to thriving.

Do not be hard on yourself for how you survived.
You made it here.
Through cracked vessels and unearthed caverns
You are here.

OUR THRIVING TOOLS

It was a typical Saturday morning. The day planned was filled with ease, containing nothing but rest. My youngest son, Jupiter, and I sat in bed, blanketed beneath the covers. There we sat watching one of his favorite kid's television shows. I don't remember the name of the show we watched. However, it involved a central animal character, sharing his and his friends' adventures. This episode was all about the different kinds of plants, fruits, animals, and even insects with shells. They mentioned the coconut and the coconut palm tree in the sand-filled islands and how tall they stood with their fruit hanging from its branches. The animal character showed how the coconut by design had a hard shell, thankfully because of its high location and its certain destiny of falling to the ground below. I sat there thinking, "Could you imagine a soft-fleshed fruit located way up in a coconut tree? It would smash upon impact, rendering itself inedible." I continued to watch as the cartoon character talked about this hard-shelled fruit, the turtle, and the snail, and how because of their soft bodies, they used their hard shell to protect themselves from their environment and surrounding predators.

As I watched, I gathered that nature, in its infinite wisdom, knew what to give each organism for its protection and thriving. Most important, we naturally have everything we need to prevail, and what we do not have, we can acquire. This chapter aims to move from our surviving tools to our thriving ones. The coconut could not have soft flesh, or it wouldn't withstand the impact with the ground, so therefore it has a shell so that when it falls, it will not break. The same is true for the snail or the turtle. When a snail or a turtle is in danger or needs a safe space, it can be its own safe space, retreating to its shell. The mantra is "We have everything we need to be and nurture our shells and safe spaces." It is by design. You are the safe space for which you've been waiting. Of course, we may need assistance such as therapy to be able to see this within ourselves.

> *Seek and find*
> *It is there*
> *All around you*
> *All around*
> *Consider the lilies.*
> *They have everything they need.*
> *As do you.*

I want you to know that feeling depressed or anxious after experiencing what seems like a lifetime of trauma makes sense. You are not broken. Your survival tool makes sense. How do we thrive after witnessing the things we've seen? How do we let go of the survival tools we relied on for so long after the danger has passed?

Thriving within our mental health requires that we switch out our toolset. Until this point, we've used the tools adapted and afforded to us for our survival. Our toolkit for thriving looks a bit different. It is rooted in sustainability as opposed to immediate settling. It is inquisitive, and, like my son Jupiter, it digs below the surface. It is not a quick fix. It is slow and steady, but when adapted proves to be long-lasting and feels a lot better in the long run. Like the coconut, we all possess thriving tools designed to keep us safe and living more abundantly, as these are the tools that provide the more long-term and healthier support we need to navigate post-traumatic events. Thriving tools are actions and rituals we use to live a life rooted in our healing instead of our trauma responses.

How do you locate your thriving tools? Our thriving tools can be modalities like yoga, therapy, or breathwork. They require us to look inward, accessing those points of safety we already possess but have yet to discover. Much like the coconut, your tools create a soft landing against the impacts of life. And one thing is for sure. Life presents challenges, as it is part of the human experience. But where do you find softness within the wreckage?

I should note that your thriving tools protect you from the impact, not from the fall itself. It is not avoidance or the fear of falling or life's hit. These new tools we put into place propel our growth and the growth of those around us. A coconut that has fallen to the ground is planted to produce another coconut tree. Your thriving tools allow your experience to be not simply that but an opportunity for yourself and others who bear witness to after and how you bloom through it. When locating your thriving tools, use these descriptors as a checklist.

SEE YOURSELF AS WORTHY

To start on your journey toward thriving post-trauma and locating your own thriving toolkit, you must first know that you are worthy. You deserve to be seen and felt, healed and whole. We must see ourselves as excellent and deserving candidates for good to happen, because we are. When I see myself blocking or sabotaging myself, I remember that my trauma will no longer hinder me from good things happening to me, but instead be a pathway and open door because of it. I am worthy. We don't see things as they are, we see them as *we* are, remember? Our response to good reflects how we see our worthiness of it and ourselves because of our experiences. We brace ourselves because trauma has taught us that we do not deserve good things. Therefore, we witness the good as we see ourselves, unworthy and borrowed. Here is where we have the opportunity to switch out our tools from survival to thriving. I will say to you as I've told myself: Because of your trauma and life experiences, who else is a more worthy candidate of receiving joy, of receiving good things? If for no other reason than your trauma, you deserve all the good and so much more. Who else is more worthy than you or I? Shifting our perspective around our worthiness can now be our thriving tool.

We must shift the way we see ourselves, our pain, trauma, and the world entangled around it. When I saw anxiety as both a strategy put in place for my survival and a result of the trauma experienced, I began to hold a lot more love for the little girl who needed to hide the knives to keep her and her family safe. I wept and held her close, celebrating her for simply making it here. Even now, I have empathy for the little girl who makes her way to the surface, attempting to protect herself by way of anxious thoughts. When this happens, I don't seek to quiet her. Instead, I assure her that the survival tool, much like an umbrella that she has picked up along the way, is something she no longer needs to keep her safe.

NAMING YOUR TRAUMA

Another thriving tool is naming your trauma and the people that played a part in its origin. This part is tricky. Because often, it is not solely the "villains" in our lives that cause lasting harm, but also the tiny cuts inflicted upon us by those we love. I wanted the heroes in my story to stay just that. As I mentioned earlier, humans are complex, layered, and somewhat complicated. We carry our trauma, trying our best to consolidate with those around us, doing the best we can. To name the trauma and its contributors, I would have to release those involved from the role I cast them in of hero or saint. Many people find themselves being a little bit of both, depending on where they are in life. I would also have to remove those involved from villains or devil and instead name them human. If I could call the people who played a part as they are, then and only then could I forgive them. One by one, I named them, evoking their names. I allowed myself to feel the anger, and then I let it go. Right there in the comfort of my bedroom. I imagined standing face to face with some and simply remembered the harm from others. I named it, felt it, and let it go. And I believe you can too. Just as I let go of the replica of myself in the cosmos, I forgave them. Trust me. It doesn't feel good to name your trauma. I felt the burning as it rose to the top of my chest. It felt like fire. So I opened my mouth, sighing out the lingering smoke as I did the grief. I screamed out the bounty of anguish and lament from a garden I did not plant. And in return, I became both steel and water. I knew both how to survive and how to love.

HEALTHY BOUNDARIES INSTEAD OF WALLS

During my therapy session, my therapist guided me in getting to the origin of my avoidance, first calling it what it was—avoidance and detachment, not boundaries. Because I felt alone and silent, I detached and avoided building relationships with my siblings. Because people hurt people, their actions cut and bruise. For me, the answer was clear: The trauma suffered by the adults in the room and my environment birthed a response of what seemed to be guarded boundaries but was in fact walls and a mile-high fortress. It was hard to allow love in, acceptance, or the shower of joy. I was at a crossroads. Either rise and grow toward the light or be swallowed up by darkness. My therapist held the mirror up, a mirror that I needed to look into, and asked, "Where are you now?"

I built a wall as a kid because I felt alone. But now, as an adult, where was I? Where was the danger now? I was no longer alone. I want you to know brick by brick. You can begin to tear down the walls, allowing people in, one at a time. Take as long as needed. There is no rush.

Listen, I love boundaries! They keep us safe within a world that can feel unpredictable and obscure. However, how do we know when we are setting healthy boundaries and when we are building walls? As I mentioned, one of the leading indicators of self-sabotage is its ability to affect one's interpersonal relationships. We shut down connections that could bring joy to our lives, all in the name of fear and our past understandings. Gentle reminder: Safe community can be one of our many thriving tools. When we build walls to avoid danger when no threat has been found, imagine if we are curiously brave enough to look at the origin of our fear and discover it is rooted in our past trauma. This understanding is how we know that our boundaries are in fact walls, embedded in our trauma and its overextended defenses. I know. It is a fine line between the two, and you may find it blurry. Consider this:

> *Boundaries are birthed from a place of observation of specific past behaviors.*
> *Walls are built from fear and may have nothing to do with fact or specific behavior.*

Boundaries are rooted in truth and the present.
Walls are rooted in fear and often the past.
Boundaries empower us to grow forward.
Walls can limit us to the past.
Boundaries often challenge us.
Walls allow us to do what feels most comfortable, cuffing us
to the familiar.
Regarding boundaries versus walls, I like to think of them
this way: Boundaries are surrounding in nature, enclosing
and protective. The healer Prentis Hemphill says boundar-
ies are the distance at which I can love you and me simul-
taneously, and I couldn't agree more. Boundaries can be
implemented, adjusted, and readjusted. Walls, by contrast,
are raised from a space of defense, often separating, and
rooted in fear, generalities, and trauma.

MINDFULNESS AS A TOOL

Let's talk about mindfulness. We hear this word tossed around in today's wellness sphere. However, the question remains, how do we implement it into our everyday life? One of the crucial things that I've discovered within healing post-trauma and practicing mindfulness is the importance of locating our present safety. After experiencing trauma, it never leaves our knowing. Remember the garlic and our nervous system? Our nervous system and brain are hell-bent on keeping us safe. Therefore, a specific smell, a distant yet familiar sound, can all trigger the ruins of trauma. And this triggered residue can leave us feeling as if we are back in the trauma. Reminder: Our brain has no sense of time when activated. Think about playing the piano. Whether you are thinking back to a time when you played the piano in the past or are playing it right now, your brain doesn't differentiate and processes it as if it is happening in the present. The same is true for triggered memories of trauma. The triggered memory of trauma sends messages throughout the body, sounding its alarm that it is happening again. We are in danger again. We are being abandoned, abused, and taken advantage of yet again. For this reason, reminding ourselves of our present safety is vital. Rooting into our present, especially when triggered, is our anchor in the here and now. It reminds us that we are not in danger. We are safe. We are not back there again. We are here.

The present is where we can unbend, straighten our back like a flower, and heal. This feeling of safety post-trauma is where we can run and find refuge when the world feels dark, unkind, and unfamiliar. After experiencing trauma, many of us find ourselves in loops and never-ending mental spirals and patterns that never seem to evaporate, as we wish they would. I want you to know that there is no magic moment, pill, or even book that can disrupt our patterns of belief that we are not worthy of safety, good things, or protection. We are the disruption that we've been waiting for. And this disruption is nothing short of an intentional choice every day of our lives to live, really live, in our present truth.

So how do we stop the spiraling? How do we implement the tools we've spoken of when triggered?

1. **We breathe.** I know, I'm bringing it back to our dear friend, our breath. However, our breath is where we find sanctuary, rest, and reminder. I've found that even when I am unsure where the trauma response train is going, taking a full deep breath in through my nose and out through my mouth immediately slows everything down. The single act of breathing will directly shift our nervous

system, sending messaging throughout our body that we are safe, even when we don't see it as so. When activated, we hold our breath, which arrests us at the current triggered moment, and the past trauma experienced. So allowing ourselves to fill our lungs with air, and exhale while sighing it out, will not only disrupt the signal that harm is near but also liberate us from the trigger response. While breathing, keep your eyes closed, as sometimes, when we are activated, everything, especially the things around us, can feel like too much.

2. **We distinguish between past and present.** While your eyes are closed, ask yourself whether it is really happening again, or is this a reminder from your nervous system that it happened? Does this feeling seem familiar? It may be a trigger or a reminder of the harm experienced. This questioning may be the first time you've traced back a feeling felt, a sense, or an emotion. However, our curiosity about the source and direction of our triggers disrupts the spiral. Ask yourself, "What is the emotion I am experiencing? When was the first time I felt this feeling?" Place your hands on your heart and hold this emotion.

3. **We take note of our surroundings.** Once you've taken a few deep breaths, open your eyes and begin looking at the things around you. Pay attention to the ground beneath you and the placement of your feet. What do you notice? Notice its similarities (if any) but pay close attention to its differences. When I would find myself triggered by loud noises in my home (which is inevitable with young children), after taking a breath, I would open my eyes and begin to notice the differences between the potting of my current environment and my childhood environment— seeing simple things such as the lush citrus trees in my

current Pasadena backyard in contrast with the home of my childhood in Alabama—and simply noticing allowed me to place my feet back into the present.

4. **We walk it out.** Moving our bodies acts as a significant disruptor of spiraling. Sometimes your body needs to move, and sitting while your brain is on a loop may not be the best. You may need to walk around your neighborhood as you breathe deeply. While walking, you can also pay attention to what you see. This movement will pull you into the present.

NEW IDENTITY

When I decided to heal, I had to begin a new identity. While what I'd been through had become a part of my story, it was just that. It's a part of your story, not who you are. You are not your trauma. As mentioned, we begin to meld into our trauma responses, forging alliances and matching them to become one. However, they are not us. So what do we do after divorcing our survival tools? We have to begin to develop a new identity, a healed identity. We have to fill those empty spaces now vacant with the things that will strengthen our healing. For example, if you find yourself flooded with energy when triggered, get up and go for a walk or a run. Move your body and that energy through. If your natural go-to survival tool (not a thriving tool) is withdrawal, get out in the sun and out in nature, allow in the sunlight. You feel isolated, do not withdraw further. Step outside, allowing your feet to touch nature, connecting with nature. You may wonder if you will recognize yourself outside of your trauma, and you may not. However, I believe that's where the rediscovery happens.

I discovered that the more I lean into the thing that my body naturally wants to resist or is fearful of, the less anxious I feel. For example, when I feel anxiety, my instinct is to freeze, a survival tool of trauma. I don't move. In my head, if I can get still enough, then the tension and fear will go away. I would equate any movement as counterproductive to my relief. I am anxious, so I fix it by "being calm." If I want to be calm, then I must be still. Freezing was how I would navigate before shifting my perspective of this overprotective friend of mine, anxiety.

One day I tried something different. The boys were running around, and the house was loud, as usual. The dog was barking. If I closed my eyes, I couldn't tell the difference between my house and WWF (kid edition). My kids would scream at the top of their lungs. Not because anything was wrong, but because they were having fun. Jon would yell from one end of the house to the other for one thing or another. With my eyes closed, all of this could sound like the foreshadowing of danger, reminiscent of my childhood, when my present reality couldn't be further from my early upbringing. However, this is what trauma does. It reminds us to be aware when we are not in danger. Forewarns us to keep watch when we can rest. It whispers for us to run and hide when there is no threat and sanctuary is present.

One thriving tool to consider when practicing mindfulness is our awareness of panic. When we are in a state of panic, we operate from a form of self-preservation. And while self-preservation is a necessary tool for survival, it is just that, to survive. We cannot flourish in a constant condition of self-preservation and fear. I correlate it to driving on a spare tire, only meant to be used in an emergency, not every day.

Affirm with me: I am available to make intentional decisions in uncomfortable conditions.

Asking ourselves the three key questions is significant, as the overall goal is to stay here and to bring our mind back to our body. The objective is to disconnect from patterns of panic, connecting us to mindfulness.

- **Who am I?** Knowing who we are right now (*not* who we were) supports keeping us planted in the present. Often our past identity can pull us back to where we begin to see the world as we were and not as we are. Past identities need not make decisions for our present selves. Remember who you are. When activated try this out: I am _____. (Who are you? What word would you use to describe the core of who you are? Are you brave? Are you safe? Triggered?)

- **Where am I?** Knowing where we're at is vital, as our experiences can teleport us back in time. We've all been there. Trauma lifts us from the ground, tossing us to and fro like the wind from one unintentional choice and action to another. Looking around and knowing where we are is a supportive tool. I hear yogis say, "Drop into your body." I like to believe it's because they also know that life can make us feel like we are floating like an untethered balloon controlled by the wind. We connect ourselves to our present reality and truth when we know where we are. Example: I am _____. (Look around. Again, glance at your feet. Where are you? In your home? At work? At the gym?) Use your senses to reacquaint yourself with the present.

- **How long have I been here?** We create a time stamp distancing us further from our past when we know how long we've been in this moment and our current reality. And when we practice mindfulness in this regard, we can shift our perspective and hitchhiker thoughts around the past.

We begin to see the distinction between the present and past and how far we've traveled to arrive safely here. And so it is. Gratitude can be birthed from this inquiry. Perhaps where you are is not where you hoped to be. Asking, "How long have I been here?" can cause us all to reflect on how long we've been in this place, prompting us to put action in motion, saving ourselves.

So what did I do on that boisterous and absolutely overwhelming day? I paused and asked myself the three foundational questions for thriving: Who am I? Where am I? How long have I been here? My answers were simple: I am safe. I am not in danger. I am in my laundry room throwing sneakers in the dryer. I am in my home. How long have I been here? I have been here for quite some time. Answering these questions grounded me in the present and snatched me right out of my past trauma and the thought of future threats.

And then I did something unusual. I went for a walk. I chose to move my body instead of freezing. As I walked around my neighborhood, I began to feel less and less stuck in my body. I felt less and less the child, without a choice, frozen in place, walking down my street, passing floral trees with the pavement below. I wasn't in the forest. However, this concrete kingdom might as well have been the woods that I explored as a child. I picked a lemon from a nearby tree. I held it between my fingers and inhaled its citrus aroma.

I continued to walk until I reached my doorstep. And once I entered my home, holding three fleshy lemons in my hands, I felt the weight of anxiety lift from my shoulders. It seemed that she left a few blocks ago, sensing that I no longer needed her. I was curiously brave.

Evolving.

Shifting.

Flowing.

You are water.

Journal Prompts

1. Name your trauma.
2. Recognize your survival tools.
3. Check in with yourself, now (Who are you? Where are you? How long have you been here?).
4. Identify your thriving tools.

CHAPTER EIGHT

Tear Down to Rebuild

Rebuilding ourselves may require us to tear down what we have known as the familiar. We humans can live and make a home out of anything, including chaos. Even though it is uncomfortable, painful even, we can adapt and live in uninhabitable places that were not meant to be our permanent space of living. I want you to know that you were not meant to live in emotionally uninhabitable spaces. While sadness is a natural emotion, living in and making a home in sadness is untenable. The same is true for anger, chaos, and the effects of trauma experienced.

A huge part of rebuilding is taking ownership of our joy. Our peace. The inner sanctuary that we've discussed in previous chapters. The knowledge that this life is truly ours to live in. My rebuilding began when I realized that no one and nothing could make me happy quite like I could. And that that happiness could finally commence right here, right now, in the present. As I began rebuilding every day, my goal was to discover new ways to make myself happy, whole, and healthy and become my first love, because I was all along. By making this decision, we can finally cease our quest for a happy ending and live in our happy right here.

After the storm of trauma, I had to intentionally decide to rebuild. The thing about this kind of healing is that the rebuilding is neither automatic nor sudden. I had to take on this objective: If I was going to heal, then dammit, let's heal it all. However long it took. Which, by the way, was a day-to-day process. Personal rebuilding has no deadline, just a long stretch of time and gumption.

And all of this took intentional work. This work looked like doing the one thing I had never done before: I had to choose myself. That meant intentionally choosing my joy, nourishment, and pleasure. All of which initially felt foreign. I was taught by trauma that I didn't matter. Neither my peace nor my safety mattered. After years of trauma, I had to intentionally prioritize my well-being and right to security, peace, and healing, never believing the lies of trauma again.

I knew I was rebuilding in this area when I began using my voice when I felt unsafe. Instead of turtling, withdrawing into the triggered response, I would speak up on how _____ made my heart, body, and spirit feel. My safety mattered, and the little girl who lacked protection was now safe, as was I. I'll never forget sitting in a workshop with Resmaa Menakem, the *New York Times* bestselling author of *My Grandmother's Hands: Racialized Trauma and the Pathway to Mending Our Hearts and Bodies*. They were speaking to a group of Black women and explained how our bodies held on to somatic memories of past trauma and why claiming our protection and safety as our own is crucial to our thriving. They shared that the simple act of walking into a space and observing the exits is not just a way of leaving in an emergency but more of a reminder that we possess full autonomy to exit any condition that feels devoid of safety, conservation, and solace. Whenever I am aware of the exits in the room, I remind myself that I do not have to remain in a place that doesn't nourish or support my rebuilding.

I knew I was rebuilding when in 2022, my family and I exited the hustle and bustle of the gritty city living of Los Angeles and found refuge within the soft foliage of Pasadena. For thirteen years, we lived in the heart of the city. Before moving to Pasadena, our last home sat on a busy street corner, where cars whizzed by from morning until the wee hours of the night. There was a constant humming that grumbled from our neighborhood's energy. Our environment was always busy, with people walking here or there, getting in and out of their cars as they too became a part of the continual buzzing I heard from the side street window.

Before rebuilding, I had always wanted to live in a bustling city. I wanted to be in the hub of it all. I really did. Until I noticed how living in such a state of nonstop activation, as sirens zoomed past, made me feel. The short answer is I didn't like it. And perhaps the hodgepodge of city living simply felt familiar and was never what I desired as home. I didn't like being on alert of what was happening next. And while we lived in a safe neighborhood, it was never quiet, always occupied, which no longer supported where or who I wanted to be. I wanted a life of softness and intentional ease. This place I had called home for so long no longer supported who I was shifting into. I wanted nature and clean air. I wanted to be surrounded by leafy plant life and nature. So we moved. We made our home in Pasadena. And it wasn't until I exited my prior environment that I instantly felt my body sigh out a big exhale. My body loosened and unwound as it let go of our previous surroundings' bound-up anxiety. Rebuilding called me to exit the familiar and enter where I knew I would have full agency to thrive.

As a Black woman and mother, prioritizing my mental health, joy, pleasure, and nourishment felt almost blasphemous. However, the mantra became *I am important. I matter.* Now I had to embody that by choosing myself. This looked like me not waiting until I was at capacity and consumed before being able to ask for help. I nurtured our beautiful boys, *and* my first priority was nurturing myself. While my children may not have known every detail of the trauma I experienced, my children saw their mama healing and whole. And this witnessing is one of the greatest gifts I can offer my children and myself.

SUPPORT AS A MEANS TO REBUILD

A crucial portion of rebuilding is support. For me, this support came by way of all types of therapy. I did talk therapy and somatic therapy. I was seeing a chiropractor and scheduling regular massage therapy. I even did physical therapy after suffering a partial muscle tear from years of holding my shoulders up to my ears. I began to notice through these various modalities how the trauma showed up in how I carried my body and, more specifically, how I walked. For as long as I could remember, I would walk on my tiptoes and not let my heels touch the ground. I would do this as a child as I would tiptoe through my childhood home, hiding all the sharp objects and listening to the adults as they fought, ready and waiting just in case I needed to spring into action. I would walk as if I were playing a game of "the floor is lava," not making a peep. I couldn't trust the floor beneath me, so I would tiptoe through the hallway, attempting to keep everyone safe. I needed the floor to not dime me out. Feet arched across the vinyl, I bargained with the floor beneath me that I would disappear into the background and the darkness, treading it lightly if I could make my rounds hiding all that could cause danger. I needed the floor to keep my secret and be my accomplice.

My tiptoeing was one of the many things that my physical therapist noticed. She would ask, "Why don't you trust the floor?" The floor was just one of many things that I couldn't trust. If I counted on it as a child, it would give up my secret, and I would for sure be in trouble for not staying out of grown folks' business, even when one of them wasn't acting like grown folks. She affirmed, "Allow your feet to touch the floor. You can trust the ground beneath you." But how could I? I'd already seen it open up from underneath me and attempt to consume me whole. How could I trust something so dual in its intentions? How could I trust something that I feared? As a child, things would be good and then terrible. Things would feel safe, and then they would quickly rearrange to the wildly unsafe.

I will share with you what I heard so loudly through our inner teacher. The floor is like the ocean. It is there to carry and hold you, not break or bury you. It is the universe. Its very role is to support you, to make all things work well for you. I knew I was on my way to rebuilding when I began practicing this brave act as I placed my heels on the ground. Even when everything within me wanted to brace myself for the floor to tell my secrets.

IT'S OKAY TO NEED MORE

I knew I was rebuilding when I finally leaned into the truth that it's okay to need more. And I want *you* to know that it's okay to need more too. It's okay if, along your journey, as your life grows and you heal, what worked for you before, now needs added support. I began medication for anxiety and depression when I, too, needed added help. And truthfully, I am hesitant to share this part of my post-trauma story, as I don't want anyone reading this to believe this is *the way* or the *only way*. In fact, it was simply one of the many ways that supported my mental health. After experiencing so much trauma, my brain needed a break from constant survival mode. I was that person who never knew of the safety that we spoke of earlier in this chapter. That was me. My brain had yet to catch up with the reality that I was no longer in danger, that I was safe. Medication served as an incredible stop-gap measure for me to finally escape the constant rut of survival. So I could utilize the thriving tools I am sharing with you today.

Will your extra layer of support be your reality forever? More than likely not. However, I want you to know that there may not be one lasting method or practice to heal but a constant evolution of ourselves and our process. I want you to know that needing more doesn't mean that the methods you implemented before within your healing work didn't take or were a waste of time. In fact, I would challenge you to witness them as steps to your current path and where you are now in your journey. It's okay to try and try again until . . . All of it is connected. Our goal is to heal by any means necessary.

VULNERABILITY TO REBUILD

To rebuild, I had to be open and vulnerable. This was the most challenging part by far. I knew I didn't want to live a life in which everything I touched was tinged with the pain of trauma. We all know people like this. They may be in your family, or your friend circle, or co-workers. People who have endured much, and the heartache, justifiable anger, and bitterness have made their home in them, rent free. Although I was in one of the darkest moments of my life, I knew there had to be an after. That there was life beyond the current pain that I felt. There had to be a place beyond the pain of now. And if I were to be so lucky to find myself in that place of whole and not battered by trauma, I didn't want what I touched to be touched by the past trauma experienced, but instead by the triumph of healing through. I had to see myself outside the trauma. Whole and, dare I say it, truly happy.

I knew that to rebuild myself to a place of wholeness and find out what kind of life was on the other side of trauma, I would have to open my hands to all that this life offered, although terrified. Closing myself off in fear of disappointment meant closing myself off from human connection and possibly healthy relationships. Closing myself off in fear of reencountering despair would disqualify me from experiencing joy. If I wanted to rebuild, I had to be vulnerable. Trust me, opening ourselves up to those around us and letting the light in can be scary, as there are no guarantees. When we vulnerably open our hands, in exchange, we can be offered a hand within our own, or a turd. However, this is the price of vulnerability. And if we want to rebuild ourselves, we must accept the unknown with the good.

Shift Your Perspective

Despite all the abuse my mother experienced, the one thing that she never lost was hope. When good things would happen, I would call her, sharing how amazed I was that I was the lucky recipient of such good fortune. She would urge me to shift my perspective, saying, "Brandi, you should expect good things." I would make a rebuttal and tell her how I never wanted to lose my sense of amazement over the good things that found their way to the doorstep of my life. She would insist, "Brandi, *you* should expect good things." Looking back, I now know that she was right. I should. We all should. Joy, happiness, and the expectation of good are all skills begging for our cultivation. Do you think the flowers don't expect the bees to come gathering and dispersing pollen from one place to another? Do you believe that they don't expect the sun to rise, providing them with light so that they can accept its caress, growing toward it? The flowers, trees, and plants worldwide and in our homes know a secret we humans have yet to discover: Nature expects to receive everything it needs to flourish and bloom.

My mother recognized that good things happen, as do the bad. And sometimes, perhaps often, we humans don't get a say. And because of this, shelter and safety feel a million light-years away, touching the stars, out of reach, reserved only for those who fate deems worthy of it. I now know that my mother was on to something. We deserve the good things that find their way home and into our hearts. And a substantial portion of rebuilding ourselves back is understanding we are worthy of good, a present not drenched in the sorrow of yesterday, and of home, so that when things begin to waver, shaking the fruit from our branches, our roots remain planted within the fortress of their soil, not breaking. Our hearts stay steadfast, holding the tree steady. And as long as we remain steady within our roots, we can always thrive and find our way.

So how do we thrive while navigating our mental health? We adopt and embrace rituals that help us feel connected to our safety and current life. And we do so by knowing and naming our North Star. Being near my grandmother's home was my safe space as a child. Safety post-trauma is wherever you can run into the arms of the here and now, taking as many breaths as you need, rocking and swaying. While our healing does not erase the past, it calls us into a gentler, softer, and oh-so-resilient present, all while dusting off our knees and tending to our wounds as a trusted elder would, so we can continue to venture out into the world joyful, despite our scars. This safety I speak of asks that we pay attention to our body's cues and the ways by which it feels displaced. Where do you feel captive within your body? Do you feel it on your shoulders? My shoulders find their own home nestled by my earlobes when I feel anxiety. They do not belong there.

I lightly take my fingers and press against the top of my right shoulder and then the left, reminding them of their true home as well. I scan my body, one part at a time, reminding each one that this moment and positioning of settled is exactly where I belong and how it is so delicious to be here. I whisper "I know," and "I love you." I kiss my hands for being brave enough to open. I take time to honor my heart for being brave enough to remain unrestricted, despite heartbreak and grief. I find this healing practice by giving love to myself. I can thank that little girl who did the best that she could by hiding knives. I can hold her and comfort her, reminding her that she is okay now. No one can snatch us away from it when we find safety within ourselves.

Forgiveness in Rebuilding

> I've learned that forgiveness is not a sign of weakness, but a strength that can heal the deepest wounds.
>
> —Maya Angelou

To rebuild, I chose to forgive those who had caused harm in my life. The funny thing about realized hurt is that it breeds anger. And while anger is neither good nor bad, it is not a place where we should live. I found that holding on to unforgiveness only made me bitter. Now, I want to be clear about what forgiveness is and is not. Forgiveness is not a sudden come-together sing-along of "Kumbaya." Nor does it mean that I have forgotten all the ways I was harmed by those in my life. It doesn't even mean I would reconnect if given the chance. Forgiveness simply means that I love myself more. I love myself more than the harm caused, the bitterness and the anger stored. And I love me so much I am willing to forgive you. Because not doing so possesses the potential of further harming me in the end. Lucky for you, I love me.

For me, forgiveness looks like this:

- I forgive those who caused me harm, whether they ever apologize or not.
- I forgive those who caused me harm, and I hope they heal the part that hurts.
- I forgive those who caused me harm, *and* I will not neglect nor ignore the wound caused by their hand.

I also had to forgive myself. I had to forgive myself for all the times I silenced my voice and downplayed the reality of what I'd experienced. And listen, I get it. Feeling what happened to us can be a weight like no other. However, we betray ourselves when we brush over our wounds in such a way. For me, self-forgiveness looked like this:

- I forgive myself for all the times that I substituted the joy of others for my own.
- I forgive myself for the time lost, not getting to know myself intimately, confiding in her, and trusting her as my closest friend, sanctuary, and confidante. I am such a good hang.

- I forgive myself for everything I didn't know before. Some things we just don't know until we do. Remember, we discover the truth when we are ready for her. So if you find yourself in the space of actualizations and the absolute heartache that follows, know that you can survive and thrive through it. My friend, remember you possess the resilience of flowers. You will flourish.

THE IMPORTANT THING

How do we rebuild post-trauma? I believe we do so by knowing two things: what's intrinsically important to us and what's the most important thing. Now, when I speak of what's essential, I'm not necessarily referencing what's important regarding our mantra or values in life overall. What I'm referring to is what's important within the experience. For example, perhaps you have an appointment at noon, and you see that you are running late. Now, if you are anything like me, I hate running behind. I hate running late, and not because I like to be on time. In fact, if I am running ahead of schedule, I will fill the time that I have nothing to do with more things if not careful. I hate running behind because of the way it makes me feel. I feel stressed and anxious, and although adequately prepared, I will suddenly begin to feel unprepared. So, in those moments, I ask myself two questions. What's important to me? And what's the important thing? What's important to me at that moment is that I not be late. So I will do what I can to be on time. However, the follow-up question regarding the most important thing is the grounder. The most important thing is that I get where I am going safely. And that once I get there, I am prepared, and I am emotionally present. The latter question allows me to zoom out and see the more comprehensive picture. My intention and goal now shift to arriving safely, being prepared, and present, and away from the fear and anxiety of simply being late. When we are unaware of what's important, our emotions and feelings can begin to feel a lot like a vagabond, searching for a place to land and grasp. Asking these questions roots us in the present, and steers us from the anxiety of the future and trauma of the past.

Identifying what's important is also vital, as our surroundings and environment communicate so many moments of having-to's, without reason or explanation. The clock reflects mile markers, ideas, and thoughts that send us whirling through an active motion to retrieve and gather what is perhaps important to many, but if we're honest, not essential to us. And so we strive toward this goal, propelling ourselves further into someone else's sense of grounding and further from our own. When we know what's important, we can silence the noise around us, which creates a further understanding of displacement and emotional vacancy.

I want you to know that it's okay if knowing what's paramount takes time to figure out. It's also okay if and when it shifts. It is okay to change your mind. Part of embodying safety post-trauma is making peace with that. It is okay that you no longer feel the same way after much research and thought. Much like the tides and the seasons, our opinions, and what's important, change. We change, as does our perspective. And when that happens, please give yourself all the permission, gentleness, and childlike freedom to tilt toward that.

THE HUMAN TRIFECTA AS A MEANS FOR THRIVING

We rebuild post-trauma by acknowledging ourselves as the complete and human trifecta that we are: spirit, soul, and body. We must find our way to nurturing all three. We nourish our body by eating meals that fill us, by moving our body, and by other health-ful practices. Getting out in nature and just walking wherever our feet take us, circulating our stagnant energy that is aching to get out. As part of reimagining my relationship with anxiety, I intentionally move it through my body one movement at a time instead of asking it to go away. I find it interesting that many of our ancestors cooked soups as tinctures for healing and health. I remember my mother and grandmother mixing herbs into broths and throwing thumb-sized pieces of ginger root, pro-nounced "ginger rut" by my grandmother, into the pot as it bub-bled and boiled. I remember the feeling not only as the soup would make its way past my lips, but as my hands touched my mother's and grandmother's and aunties' as they passed me my bowl filled with rue. Because of this, I practice the ritual of pre-paring a meal as an act of love for my body. I nourish my body not as a reward but as a thank-you for simply being here.

We nourish our spirit. We adopt spiritual practices, rituals, and ways that uplift us, building our foundation. Some of us find our way through gurus and sages, teachers and preachers. We study and find holy books, writings, and ancient scripts in foreign tongues. Perhaps for you, this spiritual work is gathering in church houses, in holy ashrams, or in the stillness and quiet. Please note that when I reference spiritual work, I am not neces-sarily referencing organized religion, as this is founded on a set group of belief systems that vary. I am instead referencing spiri-tuality, a deep linkage to what some call a higher power, some-thing expansive that connects us one to another and to a deeper understanding of ourselves. Research has shown that connecting to something or a cause bigger than ourselves can positively af-fect our mental health. Gathering together in spiritual settings can lower depression and anxiety. Studies also show that medita-tion can lower our blood pressure while enhancing brain function. Our spiritual practices connect us to ourselves, further allowing us to establish what we've talked about in previous chapters: self-sanctuary. Prioritizing a spiritual practice helps us show empathy to one another, as it brings us closer to our highest selves, reminding us that we are all connected and have challenging moments. Our spiritual path is also vital during such moments, during the hard times. Knowing that there is something bigger on our side or that we are simply surrounded by love within this life supports our mental health.

When I explore the ways by which my ancestors survived and thrived when ripped from their land, mothers and fathers, food, language, and spiritual practices, when cruel hands ripped them from their home, from the breasts of their mothers and the loving arms of their fathers, I am reminded of our deep need and yearning for that which is unseen so that we can continue to live on this side of heaven. I remember as a little girl seeing the women in our church catch the spirit, shouting and waving their arms. I remember them dancing freely as church shoe heels touched the ground and how it looked so much like the tribal dances that I was also familiar with and studied in school. I recognized that although this country had taken so much without regret, it had not taken our spirit and the ways by which it would not relent. Nourishing our hearts may look different to each individual. However, I believe that putting a practice in place, whether it be reading or praying, meditating or being still, all of this creates a pathway to seek and hear precisely what we need in all moments.

We nourish our soul. Our soul is our intellect and our mind. Much like our spirit, it is infinite and without end. We feed our soul by taking care of our mental health, seeing the therapist, and cultivating our cognitive self-care. We do the hard work that this book section is all about. We also do the small things that feed our mind, like crossword puzzles and coloring in a coloring book, slowing our brain down from the hustle and bustle and all the things we have to do. You know, all the adult stuff that presses us against the wall and pavement, at times burdening our senses, causing us to feel stuck. I love listening to storytelling podcasts. Sometimes I listen to a guest who leaves me folded forward, belly-laughing as they share the comedy of life, and other times, I am still, tears grazing my face, as I listen to the storyteller share how they, too, "got over," as the old folks used to say. Learning more about the human condition is like food to my soul. What brings you nourishment? In nourishing our soul, we are okay to do things that feel good.

SAFETY IS CALLING YOU

Affirm with me: I will provide softness where life has been hard.

Living and fully flourishing in the present—this is the gift. I no longer have to make my home inside the chaos of the past. I now go out to my backyard, pick a grapefruit from my mature citrus trees, and eat it right there as I stand barefoot in my own personal backyard Eden. Little girl Brandi is happy as a clam.

We must have the audacity to grow. It is not only the soil, sunlight, or rainwater christening the leaves and roots below that make the crops grow. It is the audacity and demand for balance between all three. To flourish, we must learn to give a kind of middle finger to anything that stands in our way of becoming, thriving, and rebuilding. I approach my continued growth and reconstruction with a sense of entitlement, as it is our birthright. It is the spirit by which we go after our healing. How entitled we are to heal our wounds and live, really live in the present, is the measure by which we will grow. What we feel entitled to is what we will pursue. If you feel entitled to good, joy, and happiness, you will develop the audacity to go after what's due you—the energy will continue to shift.

I want you to know that when you find yourself emotionally displaced, as you are looking for this "rebuilding after" or safety in the eye of the storm, this space of security desires that you find a seat within its rooms, placing your feet solidly upon its stable floor. It welcomes us and asks that we invite what's wanted into our lives, reminding us exactly where we are and want to be, here in the present. Right here, where we are free to thrive, and rest, and be, and grow. Where we are cradled in the undone and ever thriving.

So I grab my seat under my oak tree and meditate, breathing in the fresh air of my environment. And as I exhale, I am grateful that every day is another day for me to simply decide and rebuild.

1. Where are you on your rebuilding journey?
2. What are you tearing down?
3. Identify your support system for rebuilding.
4. How can you nurture your trifecta (spirit, soul, body)?

PART THREE

· ·

The Grieving Room

MARVIN, THE MUSHROOM

Mushrooms break down the dead, recycling and overturning, creating worlds and ecosystems out of that which was living. They know that even in grief, new life is possible.

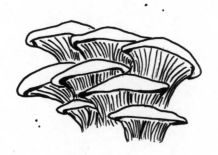

CHAPTER NINE

Sifting Through Grief

Grief arrives at our doorstep unannounced, uninvited, and without permission. It is like an unbid party guest who crashes said party without shame. Its friend, loss, preceding its arrival. Loss sits on your sofa, feet up, watching with her popcorn as the impact of her arrival unfolds, sending her unwitting and unwilling host into a timeless tailspin. By the time grief arrives, loss has made herself at home, overstaying her welcome. We want her out, and now she has invited guests into our home? Loss and grief interrupt the controlled broadcast of our lives, tossing pillows in the air, causing static and what feels like irreparable damage. It wrecks us and then leaves us in the ruins of its acts. How rude.

Just two weeks before my thirtieth birthday, my mother passed away. Unexpectedly. It was a shock that shook our family like an earthquake. However, unlike an earthquake, the earth continued to turn on her axis. I pleaded for her to pause. Not forever. Just for now. Mother Earth, she didn't listen. She continued. Being awakened by the morning sun shining through my window was an inconvenience. It was another day without her. The day-to-day task of being, let alone being asked to do anything beyond what was required, was a nuisance. Didn't they know she was gone? Didn't they—everyone—know that the world as I knew it had collapsed? I would find myself irritated by the minor things.

Anxiety, trauma, and grief danced together as I mourned the loss of my mother. She was my sun, I her earth, and much like the earth, I had to begin to soften. Open, even. I was afraid of the softening and the opening. In the months following my mother's passing, I cried so much that I googled whether one could run out of tears. I found out that one cannot. I read that there is a vast difference between tears' chemical makeup that brings moisture to your eyes and those born out of sadness. FYI, "sad tears" are filled with toxins that desperately need release. After crying, I would feel so much better, if that were possible. After a "good cry," my voice and breath would shake, eventually resolving to a slow and steady pattern. I had this fear that if I allowed myself to fall into the ocean of tears, my emotional boat would break and perhaps become shipwrecked and forever lost. I was heartbroken. How could I be so sure that this act of opening wouldn't also crush my bones and grind them into dust? The sun would continue its dance of rising and setting. I didn't want to feel. I also didn't want to break. Foolish, perhaps, but I assumed that two or three months would be plenty of time to pick myself up and brush off the yuck of loss. Although the first month after, I was in total shock, feeling nothing. I was a shadow lingering in the corners of this world. I had assumed that my grief would be different, easier, and maybe nonexistent because there was no uncleared air between my mother and me. That somehow I wouldn't feel the blunt force of heartache. I was wrong.

During my late twenties, my mother was diagnosed with cancer, but as the years went on the cancer went into remission and we mostly assumed that she was on the upswing. My mother suffered from cancer for three years before succumbing to it. No one else in our family had ever contracted the horrible disease. She was diagnosed in 2009, just a few months after Jon and I decided to make the cross-country trek from Nashville, relocating our family of three to Los Angeles. Until then, I'd lived only a couple of hours away from my mother for almost ten years. To finally move thousands of miles away and discover months later that my mother had cancer was horrific. I couldn't digest the news. I repelled the truth, as it was too bitter to taste. My mother was sick, but she would be okay. She had to be. This woman had been kicked and bruised by life and what, at some point, she thought to be love. And yet she was as shiny as an unscratched coin. Indeed, cancer was no match for her brilliance. Just as she had beaten many things before, in my mind, my mother would beat this too. My mom and I talked every day. Not a day went by that we did not commune. Imagine my surprise when the phone calls stopped. After diagnosis, my mother underwent treatment. Between chemo and radiation, both in-state and out-of-state at the cancer treatment facility, it seemed as if she would pull through. I still remember her calling me to tell me the good news. Hope had returned. I could hear it in her voice as she screamed excitedly into the phone. The cancer was gone. All of her trying to survive had worked. However, in year three, it seemed some part of the sickness had resurfaced, and this time, it was relentless and ferocious, the way it wanted to take her, my mother. I knew something was off. I denied it. I was still trying to figure out life, new parenthood, and where my pending aspirations fit in the midst of it. My stepfather had begun to answer her phone when I called, saying she was busy.

I should have known then. I would assure myself that if some-thing were wrong, my parents would surely tell my sister and me. In this case, going against my gut would prove to be an act of treason. My mother and I had never gone weeks without communicating; it had been three weeks since our previous con-versation. Our last chat had felt odd and stagnant, lacking the fluidity of the millions upon millions of conversations shared be-tween my mother and me. Our talk lacked the silly dialogue often present between us. I listened to her muttered words, misplaced and unrecognizable. My mother's voice, which often rose with excitement, didn't ascend beyond a faint whisper this time. She was weak, and I could hear it in her voice. "Jax is start-ing first grade next year." She'd repeat similar surface sentences during our exchange, when usually nothing was ever surface be-tween us two. We were as deep as the womb of the ocean. And for the first time, our words lay just above the waves, washing themselves further and further from shore. Three weeks later, my stepfather called and asked if I could come home. I had so many questions.

I do not recall whether I took the liberty to ask any of my questions or just continued to listen for any indication that life was about to change. My stepfather gave limited information. He mentioned that my mother had left the hospital and some-thing about a sinus infection. His voice felt hurried and dis-jointed. There was something beneath the surface. A voice I had never heard before. Ronald was unsettled. I listened for clues as to why I hadn't heard high or low from my mother. Why she'd felt distant when I spoke to her the last time. And why she was now silent and couldn't come to the phone. I wanted him to tell me if there was something wrong. If my mother was in danger or sick again. He didn't say. "Come home," he said.

And with those words, my body froze, a trauma response I

had felt too often prior. However, this time I didn't see the danger before me. It was all intuition and guessing and imagining the worst-case scenario. And even with this mental forecasting and preparation, I still wasn't prepared for what I would encounter upon my arrival. There was no mention of cancer ravaging her body and leaving her incapacitated. There were no words and yet all the words. I was too afraid to ask the questions bellowed by my intuition. In mid-June, Jon and our then five-year-old eldest son, Jax, packed our bags. I remember us all getting on the plane to Birmingham and feeling in my gut that something, perhaps everything, was wrong.

Upon my arrival at my parents' home, family members greeted me, preparing me for what I would see as I entered my parents' bedroom. I walked through the foyer. Everyone was present, aunties and uncles, cousins and grandmother. The only thing missing was the fireflies that fluttered so very effortlessly through our childhood skyline. Everyone was present except my mother. Where was she? When my family would entertain, you could always find my mother scurrying around and either putting something in the oven or taking something out. She would stand in her kitchen, hand on her hip, laughing, engaging, and drawing you in with her big brown eyes.

My father took me, my sister, stepsisters, and stepbrother downstairs into the den of their home, before seeing my mother. He explained to us that cancer had returned hard and fast. That it had spread to my mother's brain and that there was nothing more that the doctors could do. Dad explained that the only option left was a clinical trial or a surgery that had the possibility of rendering my mother vegetative. The room stood still as the tears welled but wouldn't fall. My eyes felt like clouds holding my tears close, suspending them from dry land in much need of saturation. The room felt tiny and began to get even smaller as

Ronald continued with the heartbreaking news. Everything was wrong—all of it. My mother wasn't okay.

That night, as I walked into her bedroom, her face lit up, and her voice made some intelligible sounds. There she was in a hospice-approved hospital bed. Cancer had spread to her brain, disabling her ability to speak or move with the agility that my mother could previously. She attempted to sit up. I could tell that she was surprised by my arrival. I fought back the tears as I searched desperately for a chance to laugh with her again. I hugged and kissed her as I held her hand, tracing the lines within them. I'll never forget the touch of my mother's hands. They held comfort and joy, soft like cinnamon butter. Visitors would enter and leave. Hospice would come in to bathe her. I and others would feed her. I would tell her over and over again that I loved her. So much so that one time, she became annoyed and formed the words "I know." I laughed because although my mother was in tremendous pain, in and out of consciousness due to her medica-tion, I now knew that she knew that I loved her. And by the im-mense effort that it took for her to form her lips to say the words "I know," I knew that she loved me too. I saw my mother peering through the fog of it all and I could tell that she saw me for a split second. This experience is how I found out that my mother was dying. There was no chance for goodbyes or conversations missed.

I spent three weeks with my mother, sitting by her bedside, and afterward returned home to California. Here's the thing about death, even when it appears unmistakable. When it comes to our parents and others we love, it's difficult to accept death's pending arrival. I went back to California unsure of when I would return. I was in denial. My mother would be okay, I thought. I kissed my mother's forehead before leaving her bed-room and heading to the airport. She looked at me as if to say, "I'm tired. Please believe what you see in front of you." I couldn't.

My lips whispered "I love you" for what seemed to be the millionth time in three weeks. I would be back, I promised, as I made my way to the airport, back to Los Angeles. I hugged my stepdad, affirming my return. However, I didn't know when. In my head, although all signs pointed otherwise, I just knew that my mother would pull through. She had already experienced so much in life. So much that perhaps could have killed her long before cancer should have. She had survived an abusive lover, my father. If she could survive that hurricane of a soul, she could survive anything.

I remember looking at my stepfather and saying the words "I'll be back when . . ." The end of the sentence escaped me. When does one come back after visiting their terminally ill parent? When does one return after seeing their parent in hospice care? My mother would survive this, and I would be back in a few weeks. By then, my mother would be back on the upswing. I would come back home, and there she would be in her usual bed. Not her hospital bed. Eyes bright and full of life. She and I would talk more about thread counts, strawberry picking, and her Christmas decorations thoroughly planned out in advance for the holidays. My mother was not dying, and perhaps that's why I couldn't finish the sentence about when I would return.

My stepfather would call me with the same voice, still unsettled and still distant, asking me to return. He didn't tell me why. Looking back, I don't believe he could utter the words for himself and for me. It was too hard. Moments later, through a group text thread he had forgotten to delete me from, while in the airport restroom, I found out my mother was gone. I boarded the plane. I sat in my seat and sobbed while buckling my seatbelt before takeoff. My mother was gone.

· · · · · · · · ·

On my thirtieth birthday, I asked a few friends to go bowling. I wouldn't say I liked bowling. Honestly, wanting to go bowling should have been a clear indication that I wasn't okay. It had only been two weeks since my mother's transition. I remember getting all dressed up, wearing sequins and a heavy smoky eye. I wore six-inch heels to a bowling alley. Perhaps I believed that by looking put together, I could mask my grief. I rolled the ball down the lane, hyperfocused. I was both numb and dolled up. Disoriented and ill-prepared like many when life does what it does. Much like the bowling pins in front of me, the present time stood still. I could hear the conversations from the nearby lanes. I listened to the rumbling of the bowling balls being thrown forcefully by fellow patrons. Did the pins ahead know that as sure as they stood, a gigantic bowling ball was heading hard and fast in their direction? Did they prepare? I didn't. Like them, I felt as though my feet had been knocked right from underneath me, landing me firmly on my ass. *Why am I here?* I asked myself. My birthday guests watched as I rolled the ball down the lane.

Smile. No tears. Smile again. Strike. The bowling pins collapsed, much like I so desperately wanted to. I didn't want to be there. Perhaps the constant sound of gutter balls and pins falling was better than the deafening silence of grief felt at home. I wasn't ready to sit with the reality that my mother was no longer with me. The thunderous sound of bowling balls crashing to the floor and rolling down the lane felt better. And the smell of bowling alley French fries, a greasy temporary relief to my wounded soul.

There's not a day that goes by in which I don't think about my mother. There will never be a day when my mother's passing will be okay with my soul. Allowing myself to crack open like a seed, exposing the delicate parts, dismembered, sad, and yet still be alive. How was it possible that I could feel this heartbreak, this pain, and feel joy again at some point in my life? How was it possible that I felt empty, depleted, and dried out from all the tears that watered my pillowcase? Yet here I was, present.

During my grief, if I were a plant, my leaves would have appeared dry and brittle. I would have been in desperate need of sister sun's rays or a drink from a nearby river. In my grief, I would get my period two times per month. My womb was telling me to slow down. To cry it out. I began taking yoga classes a few times a week, along with acupuncture. After one yoga class, the song "Girl on Fire" by Alicia Keys played. As the song bellowed, tears fell down my cheeks. I was showing up for myself. I was tending to my garden, dry leaves and all. My mother was now one with the earth—body to soil. Perhaps now she was a part of a tree, deeply rooted and intermingled with the ground.

Cry if you want to.
Yell
Scream
and kick
It's your grief, and you can grieve how you want to.
There are no rules for grief or a broken heart.

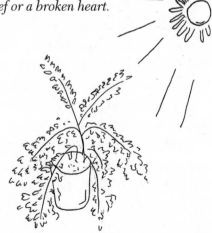

Grief and its care remind me of my maidenhair fern, Minnie. I purchased her from a local plant shop after attending a birth. I was drawn in by her delicate leaves, which resembled snowflakes. This fern looked different from the previous ferns that I had purchased. Instead of the long spear-like body of the Kimberly fern, this maidenhair fern reminded me of the paper doll cutouts holding hands that we created as children in elementary school. This plant was stunning and yet so very fragile in many ways.

Initially, I put Minnie in a secluded corner of our home. I hoped that the growth that she experienced in the plant shop would continue. Usually, when I shop for plants, I pay close attention to their plant shop surroundings and ask as many questions as I can think of before leaving to ensure that when the plant comes home with me, it experiences the least amount of shock. Minnie's plant shop home was in a shadowed place. So it would stand to reason that I would put her in a shadowed place in my home to replicate her former environment. However, I would eventually find out that that same type of environment no longer suited her upon entering my home. Minnie began to wilt. I then moved her to my bright and airy kitchen. I read that maidenhair ferns enjoyed the sun. My avocado-colored eating space with its bright and sunny windows felt like the perfect place. It was not. The sun scorched her delicate lacelike leaves, burning them to a crisp. As I swept up the brittle pieces of Minnie, my mind churned with curiosity. Of course, I researched more as I became more and more invested in the longevity of this plant. I wanted her to survive.

I understood that her transition of what she called home more than likely felt sudden and brutal. Perhaps even as sudden as the loss that I experienced in my own life. However, I needed her to be human and tell me what in the hell she needed. I considered putting her in the bathroom much like I did my Kimberly fern and peace lily whenever they needed a bit of moisture, my thought process being that ferns like water and hate being dry. Where's the best place in my home for humidity? The bathroom.

I moved Minnie into our bathroom, where she would begin to die another thousand deaths. By this time, all that was left of Minnie's leaves were ten of her original stems. I'm convinced that if she were a human, she would at that point have resembled Samuel L. Jackson in Spike Lee's *Jungle Fever*, a struggling crack addict. She was barely hanging on and a shadow of her former self. I began to think, "Does this plant even want to survive?" It for sure seemed as if she didn't.

There was one last place that I could put her. I hoped that perhaps the same magic that I had worked for my palm (about which you will hear in chapter 12), I could evoke for her. I remembered being out and about and spotting a maidenhair fern at a local park gathering. This fern was just out in the bright sun. When I saw it, I was confused, as I had read that these ferns were so vulnerable and that space in not so direct sunlight was best for this particular plant. Seeing this plant basking in the sun proved that my first impression of replicating her familiar environment was inaccurate. For the new space that she was in, Minnie needed the sun for this level of shock. So I attempted putting Minnie in a moderately sun-filled window again, this time out of the kitchen and in a north-facing window. I'm not sure why this north-facing window worked, as opposed to the kitchen window. It just did. I gave her a good gulp of water and walked away. One by one, her leaves began to emerge. She started to resemble the plant I fell in love with at the local plant store. This growth continued for a week or two. Minnie and I were on a winning streak, and no one or nothing could stop us now.

Then a heat wave struck Los Angeles. It was August or September, and the heat rolled through our city, taking no prisoners and producing exhaustion and the desire and need to stay cool. Minnie began to wilt again. The sun scorched her delicate leaves. What had been green and thriving began to crisp again into crunchy brown leaves, falling to the floor as if to wave the white flag and surrender the battle finally. Why was this happening? What worked for her survival previously was no longer adequate but now antiquated. Her transition to our home from her former plant shop shelving needed more sensitivity and awareness in navigating this significant change. The changes that Minnie was experiencing during such a great location transition required more than a textbook on how to deal and thrive when one's world is uprooted and thrown into the unknown. She needed flexibility and gentleness to flow with her day-to-day needs because when experiencing such a shift, all one can do is simply take it day by day.

I, too, felt uprooted and snatched away from my home. I felt the aching in my chest that one can only experience with such a loss. During the first year, I would sit in my car watching people walk by. The year of firsts was the most challenging and carried what seemed to be the heaviest load of grief. These were tough: the first holiday, the first birthday, the first full trip around the sun. The year of firsts after loss all serve as reminders of the audacity of life's continuance and the tragedy that it pauses for no one, not even the brokenhearted. I would sob and wonder if it would be weird for me to ask one of these strangers to wrap their arms around me and hold me close. The strangers would usually be middle-aged women with what looked like kind and inviting smiles. I watched them as they passed by. Some of them with their children. Most of them alone. I saw one woman who looked as though she gave the best hugs. Her shoulders were broad, her chest and belly soft. I didn't know her, but I imagined myself getting out of my car, walking up to her, and not even having to ask for a hug. Instead, she would just know that I needed my mother, or any mother figure for that matter. And perhaps for just sixty seconds, this intimate stranger could fill the void of isolation that I felt. I was only thirty years old. No one in my circle knew what it felt like to have a parent leave this earth. I was so very surrounded. I was also so very alone.

I became afraid of the loneliness. I felt so outside of my body that I imagined the grief consuming me and that I would never return to my former self again. I imagined going away. Not forever, but just so that no one would see me so broken, displaced, and far from home. I considered the possibility of committing myself and imagined white padded walls surrounding me so as not to disrupt the already disrupted. This heartbreak couldn't be ordinary. This despair that filled my chest with so much grief, so that I couldn't even breathe, couldn't be what others who had experienced such loss felt. I wanted the sadness to fade into the background.

In the barren land
Where there is no sun
Where there is no rain
You are the maker and can bloom there too.

After much trying to make it end, the pain was still there. I tried everything. I attempted acupuncture, yoga, and praying it away. After trying and trying, I realized that the pain of loss would forever be present. And perhaps that, too, is a gift. To grieve means that you have had the privilege of relationship. To grieve is proof that you have had the opportunity to love and to be loved. When the pain didn't go away, despite all of my efforts to make it do so, I realized that it was perhaps present for a reason and that it, too, served a purpose.

Was there a moment where I simply knew or had an aha moment? Not so much. After six months or so of playing dodgeball with grief, I just became tired. I was exhausted from running, avoiding, and trying to do a rush job of suturing the brokenness together as if the loss had never happened. I became weary of burying my grief because it was too painful to fully feel. What we resist persists.

I was tired. Are you? The tears were a reminder of love and how it transcends time and space, heaven and earth. We can carry love in all of its manifested forms. No matter how painful.

Heat Waves of Grief

How do we thrive while experiencing grief and loss? We hold and comfort our pain. We cradle it and have respect for it. I would ask that you not judge or label it. I would ask that you try your hand at allowing it to be as is, a reminder. Our grief is an intuitive reminder or teacher of the healing needed. As with anything that has been broken, we must be aware of it. Much like my maidenhair fern, for whom the brightly lit windowsill worked until it did not. The same is so while grieving. You hear that grief comes in waves. I like to say that grief comes like a sunburnt heat wave, perhaps out of nowhere and unexpected, burning you to a crisp and leaving you crumbled on the floor. And because it comes in waves, what worked for you in the beginning process of loss may no longer work for you in the present moment. It's about survival, paying attention to what's working now, not what worked before the loss or even yesterday. If I had kept Minnie on the windowsill after experiencing the scorching heatwave, simply because that's what had seemed to help her thrive before, she would have died. The same is true for us while grieving.

After my mother's passing, I tried to continue as usual. I picked up our regular schedule as if nothing had happened. I shot a music video one month afterward. I would drop Jax off at school as always. After which, I was quickly reminded that the normalcy that I craved was now altered. My mother and I would talk on the way back from dropping Jax off at school. And now my morning car talks were no more. My world was now different, and not knowing when and if the heat wave of grief would hit was exceptionally hard. However, much like Minnie, I had to learn to change my position or placement if I wanted to survive.

If we are looking to thrive during grief, we again must take a cue from the seed process. We can learn from its operation when we consider the seed and all it endures to germinate and become. As mentioned earlier, for a seed to grow into a thriving plant, it must go through the process of more than just photosynthesis. It must have a viable living environment and nutrients. A dear friend and botanist, Dr. Tanisha Williams, refers to the seed as a baby with a backpack when it sets out on its journey of germination. When it begins on its way to growing, it has everything it needs to survive the torrential road ahead. When I think of thriving through the grief process, I like to compare it to the operation of seed dispersal known as endozoochory. Dr. Williams describes endozoochory as a form of scarification, a method seeds use to move around and grow if all goes well. For the most part, all sorts of wildlife play a role in this process.

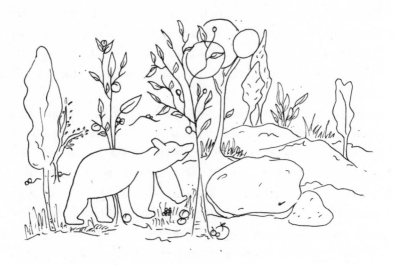

Imagine that an animal foraging through the forest, noticing a soft fleshy fruit, gobbles it whole, without disrupting the seeds within. The seeds make their way through the digestive system of the animal. The animal's stomach acids do their job by creating just enough scarification of the top layer of the seed to aid in the germination process so that the kernel itself can break through its otherwise hard shell. What should be noted is that although scarification happens, the seed is strong enough and has developed protection against digestion by the animal, thanks to its tough seed coat. The very thing that protects the seed is the same thing that needs to be cracked open for its growth.

Once the seed makes its way through the animal's digestive tract, it is pooped out. And there the seed remains, in the shit. I'm sure that while sitting in shit is perhaps not a place most of us would enjoy, it is the perfect place for the seed to grow after it has endured such a wild and arduous experience. Eventually the shit breaks down and becomes fertilizer, aiding in the flourishing of the grain. And there, within the stink of it all, the seed breaks free, begins to germinate, and grow.

So many of us feel swallowed alive, buried deep within the belly of sadness, sorrow, and heavy loss of grief. Within the belly of the beast that is grief, I imagine that much like us, the seed doubts it will survive, let alone thrive. The acidic taste of mourning burns us as we make our way through the process of loss. A burning fire, torching our dreams of what we hoped and lost alongside that which is missed. Our hearts burn for what was lost, and what we believe can never be rekindled. Once grief has had its way with us, it shits us out. I remember feeling alone in my shit. Part of me wanted to be alone. I felt shame that my heart had broken in such an intense way. I wanted to be stronger, or at least to appear so. However, how strong can one possibly look while covered in shit?

Thriving during a loss is sitting in the dung of grief, knowing that the dung is also fertilizer. The more I tried to present as more robust, more together, or less sad, the more I would find myself right back where I started. There was no progress. Could you imagine the seed after getting shat out, announcing to the world, "Nope, this shit is not for me? I'm leaving." It would not survive if it walked away from this imperative process. And more than likely it would be swallowed up again, never to emerge this time around. The same is true for the grieving process. We have to feel it to heal it. Again, grief is the most incredible reminder that we encountered love.

Grief is a lifelong process. I say lifelong because grief is as transient as nature, coming and going as it pleases, usually abruptly announced in the form of reminders. A reminder can be a song, a smell, or a phrase spoken by a stranger. What do we do when we are reminded? And how do we not stay in the abyss of mourning, a place that is neither good nor bad, but instead, somewhere between before and after, and what we must experience in exchange for our thriving? There was a time that everything reminded me of my mother. There are moments when it still does. I am reminded when I see people with their mothers shopping for towels. My mother loved hunting for washcloths, towels, and bed linen. In my early twenties, she would drag me kicking and screaming into the local Bed Bath and Beyond. At twentysomething, I couldn't understand her appreciation for towels. Like her love for gardening, towels, too, were a puzzle to me. However, my mother and I would have some of our best conversations wandering through the aisles of the bedding store. She would laugh, as I'm sure she'd purposely stretch out our time together in the store. She'd explain the difference between thread counts and why certain sheet sets were better than others. I would roll my eyes and giggle as she caught my tepid response at her enthusiasm.

After her passing, I remember walking through the bedding store and seeing mothers and daughters shopping for towels, laughing and giggling. Eyes would roll between them too. I'm sure the daughter had yet to fully understand the importance of having a good set of towels, the value of her mother's words, and just how fleeting the moments are between the two of them. Initially, I'd feel the grief rolling in. The anger grew as I was reminded that I would never experience this moment again with my mother. I'd fight the urge to go over to the mother and daughter, begging the younger of the two to be present and perhaps care. Grief at that moment would remind me of what was no longer present. However, after allowing the sadness to show up in whatever form it presented itself, I let the grief serve as a reminder that I had had the privilege of experiencing such a profound mother-daughter relationship. I began to thank heaven and earth that while there was so much more I could have said to my mother, there wasn't much of importance left unsaid. There were no bridges uncrossed or unmended. And if I could only hold on to these few statements to envelop and nurture my way through, then that's what I was going to do. I was going to hold on.

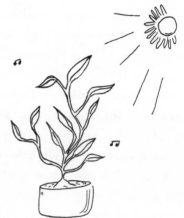

Dark clouds do not stay.
Rain showers do not stay.
Water pours from the clouds,
   watering the earth.
It leaves, although one day it
   will return.
Rainbows come.
Joy cometh in mourning.

IN THE SHIT

So what is the work that we do while sitting in the shit? What does it involve? You and I both know that it's not enough to sit in the armchair of grief. How would we not become entirely consumed by it? We must first recognize the reality of grief, all of its welcome and unwelcome friends, and, most important, what's not needed while finding our way through. Shame on its own is not required in the process of loss. It serves no one to run ourselves through the wringer of what we didn't do or what we could have done more of. Shame is the equivalent of a child lifting a thousand-pound weight. The load is too heavy, and no one can handle the endless cycle of ruminations to which it leads. When we become stuck in a loop of shame and guilt, we rob ourselves of the present-day reality and fruitlessly relive what we can't change of the past.

Shame also prevents us from accepting not only the love that we had in our heart for what was lost, but perhaps the love reciprocated, causing us to feel unworthy of our healing and journey forward. Shame is blinding in that way, and if not accompanied with the truth, it can be a roadblock to our newly bloomed selves. We must arm ourselves with reality, as mentioned in earlier chapters. When we feel the darkness of shame imposing on us, whispering subtly of how we fell short or weren't enough to stop, fix, or see the inevitable, we must remind ourselves of the truth. I suggest constructing columns and listing the ways in which you feel ashamed, knowing that shame is simply fear expressed. What are the facts to counter the shame?

Guilt is the same. When we experience loss of any sort, we try to reason with it, explaining why something so complex is happening and how we can tame its storm. We insert ourselves, proposing that we could have stopped the loss from happening when we all know that we don't possess that level of control. I was not present when my mother drew her last breath. And for a while, I felt guilt and shame around my absence. I would beat myself up and question how I couldn't know that she was dying. Before she transitioned, I stayed by her side for almost three weeks.

When we enter into grief, our bodies provide the gift of shock, protecting us from feeling what we are not yet ready to absorb. I know full well that had I taken in what was happening with my mother, if I had known entirely that my mother was transitioning in such a sudden way, my body would have collapsed. The weight would have been too heavy to carry. After her passing, I would feel guilty that I didn't stay. Guilt that I didn't allow the reality of what was happening with or without my consent to set in so that I could say a proper goodbye, adorn my mother with more

I-love-yous and more thank-yous. However, shock presented itself and thereby also saved me and my sanity. Shock knew in her infinite wisdom that I would allow the reality to wash over me when I was ready. I could continue to beat myself up, to ruminate over what I would have done if I had stayed longer and witnessed my mother take her last breath. Or I could thank my body for having the intelligence to protect me at that moment.

Another part of sitting in the shit is knowing that there are no rules to grief. There is no rhyme or reason for the mystery of emotions that one experiences after loss. Grief is a lot like people, both complicated and layered. You do not have to make your sorrow or expression thereof make sense, as they may not.

There is also no time limit on grief. There is no time limit on anger or sadness. One of the best things we can do while sitting in the shit is to allow ourselves to be as messy and weird as we need to be. Grief shows up in many forms. For example, when experiencing loss, one may feel anger, confusion, longing for control, and yes, shame and guilt. And because of this, guidance and support are vital. It takes soil and shit, earthworms, water, and so much more to grow your favorite plant life. One modality alone is not enough to sustain the plant. To support the waves that arrive during our grief, we must couple our anger with therapy and our should-haves with the truth. Give yourself all of the things you need.

Grief is one of life's great labors in which we don't have a say when entering it. We are just tossed into it, like being thrown into the swimming pool's deep end, never having swum before, hoping to paddle instinctively and make it out alive. And because of this, once we find ourselves there in the middle of the pool, flopping around for dear life, we must make the conscious choice to COME into grief:

Community (allow it to show up for us as we are wading)
Open (in grief; be open to whatever comes up for us, both
ugly and pretty)
Move (move the suffering through our body)
Ease (it is the gift we give ourselves during grief)

Community saved me during grief. It looked like friends I could call and hold the phone in silence, as my words stayed lodged within the origin of my throat. I had a friend who, too, had experienced the loss of her mother at an early age. She consented to my calling her anytime, day or night. I called her when challenging moments were present, and she assured me that (1) I wasn't losing my mind, I just really missed my mother, and (2) this, too, would pass. And not necessarily the grief around my mother's passing, but more so the intense day-to-day heaviness of it. This grief buddy system is not meant to take the place of therapy, but to act as an additional resource for support.

Openness for whatever comes up within your grieving process. This part was especially hard for me. As one who had already experienced trauma, the surprising nature of grief was an unwelcome visitor. One day I was okay and doing backstrokes like a pro, and the next, I'd be doggie paddling and sinking to the bottom of grief. Every day was different. I found that the more I tried to control and fight against the waves of grief, the more I would sink as opposed to swim. I had to become open to this secret: that I was not in control of how this grief would appear. I had to remain open to each day being different from the last. I had to change my phrasing from good or bad days to my current grief-filled days. Because truthfully, even though I had a tear-free day, I was still in the thick of loss. Where was I? Grieving.

Move the grief through your body. I've found that grief can feel stuck in our body, aching to get out. This stagnation may manifest physically and emotionally to the point where you feel yourself floating unhoused within your body. It's essential that during grief, we stay connected to our body and remind ourself that we are still here and there is a place and available container to hold all parts of ourself, even the heavy load of loss. Yoga helped me release the waves of grief. Bending and arching would almost immediately release the dam of tears that so desperately needed to come forth. Even now, years later, after experiencing the loss of my mother, dancing around my kitchen almost instantly moves the grief through, allowing it to show up and find its freedom.

Ease and rest were a sweet salve as I mourned the loss of my mother. The ways by which I would push myself to proceed without regard for how I was feeling before grief had no place here in the land of loss. There was before loss and after loss. And in this time of after, I required a more peaceful life. More empathy. More ease and tenderness. In this space, I held myself in a comforting way I never had before. If I needed to stop, I stopped. When I could go forward, I did. I communicated with those around me my need for more ease. So if I needed to postpone a meeting or a previous commitment, many understood. Things were different. And I was finally ready to sit with it.

Your grief doesn't have to be refined or dignified. It doesn't have to be wrapped up in a bow and presentable. Also, much as the seed's temporary home of shit eventually becomes fertilizer, providing nutrients to the source and the soil, the grieving process is just that, a process. Trust and respect the process. And much like any process, it is temporary. Every day, ask yourself, "What do I need, at this moment, to feel okay?" And while I don't advocate for substitutions to avoid feeling what you feel, I do, however, want you to know that you can give yourself what you need to feel okay. Healing is a lot of work, and during grief, you reserve the right to take a break from work so that you can jump back in when you are ready. Healing is not about weighing ourselves down with more things to do, but about adding a foundation beneath our feet so that we can continue through. This foundation feels soft and looks like connection with those around us and the allowance of nurturing. Trust me, it's easier said than done. Especially if you are usually the one doing the nurturing. In gathering, we are surrounded in love, while steeped in emotional chaos and grief.

Sitting in the shit of grief involves knowing that once the gift of shock subsides, you are more than capable of withstanding its aftereffects and stench. Much like the seed, you have survived being swallowed alive and the acidic process of loss. Your topcoat, although scarred, has made it easier to be cracked open so that you can bloom, and that cracking open has gifted you with empathy and an awareness that one might otherwise never experience (until it is their turn). It wasn't until I felt the pain of loss that I understood and saw what my friends who had experienced the loss of a loved one had moved through. Going through my digestive process of grief cracked my heart wide open for all pain experienced. And because of that, I can see just how connected we humans are within the watering of our tear-filled gardens. We are connected by grief, and because of it we are never entirely alone.

1. Grief comes in waves. When in the room of grief, explore how it is requiring you to move differently.
2. The shit is the doorway through grief. What does the shit look like for you?

3. Is shame or guilt showing up in the shit for you? Identify the areas where shame is taking place. What are the counteractive facts?

4. Joy cometh in mourning. How are you experiencing joy and mourning simultaneously?

CHAPTER TEN

Death—the Start, Not the End

The year 2012 was the pits. Greg, my birth father, died tragically in a house fire six months after my mother's death. I received the phone call from my stepdad, Ronald, who had received the news from my grandmother. This particular morning, Ronald's first words were, "Are you driving?" I was. I'd just dropped off Jax at school, and was beginning my drive home. I was already steeped in mourning, and the missing of the morningtide call with my mother and receiving this kind of call felt like an overbearing rush of wind that could officially knock me to the ground. Ronald asked that I pull over. I did. And then he shared with me the news that Greg, my father, was dead.

My initial guess was that the fire was self-inflicted. Greg had engaged in his fair share of suicidal ideations and attempts at ending his life throughout my childhood. He was no stranger to entertaining or even pursuing the thought of ending his life, and by default, neither were the people closest to him, dealing with the repercussions of his self-destructive tendencies.

After my parents split, I remember our last after-school visit.

It was just he and I in our neighborhood park, surrounded by wilted orange and brown leaves crunching beneath our feet. The air was crisp and cold. The autumn trees looked on as we sat on the park bench together. I had worn a button-up cardigan to school that day, more than likely with a turtleneck as a protective layer, warding against the vulnerability and perhaps harm of the cold, cold air. After ten-plus years, my mother had finally found the strength to leave Greg. I was ten years old and had more than likely seen more backhands to mouth, bloody lips, and screams in the night by this time than most children my age. This particular day, he surprised me, picked me up from school, and took me to a park.

Truthfully, I'm not sure if he was supposed to pick me up or not. My mother, in her protection of my sister and me, and herself, did not allow visitation. The truth is, my mother fled with us. She packed our bags quickly one afternoon, loaded us into her car, and we left to live with my grandmother. We returned only once to gather forgotten items. I returned with my mother, my shoulders raised to my ears and stomach in knots. My mother didn't seem to be afraid. However, I was. As a child, my father's mere presence, accompanied by his unpredictable moods, produced a wave of instability that by default created unmatched fear without his uttering a word.

I think that my mother wanted my father to see her face as she took back her power and walked freely out the door, something that she'd perhaps wanted but had lost the courage to do over and over again so long ago. I stood there with my mother, clutching her hand tight, hoping that my little fingers would meld into her adult hand, protecting, shielding, and perhaps disappearing me from what could happen next. As a child, I wished over and over to become like the great magicians and simply disappear. Nothing happened as my mother walked away with my sister and me. Greg's tall and skinny frame sat on his upholstered La-Z-Boy sofa, drink in hand. He sat there calmly, almost as if my mother's threat, and now realized departure, had conjured a spell above all spells, freezing him in the space and not allowing him to move from his upholstered throne. He glared at my mother, and then at me, and then at my sister. We were then ten and two years old. And although he didn't raise his hands to punch or slap, his words did just as much damage. My father insisted that he never wanted to see me again if I left. He dismissed me as no longer his daughter and bade me good riddance with those words. My father suffered from undiagnosed mental illness. And while I know that he didn't mean the words that exited his mouth, they felt like the emotional grave that preceded his physical one.

I don't even remember how Greg and I arrived at the park that frigid fall day. My mind remembers only my father and me sitting on the park bench, just us two. I'd recently learned how to construct a makeshift stovetop using a large can in my Home Economics class. Before our time together, I suppose I had coerced my father into witnessing my new skill. I proudly presented to my father what I had learned while cooking pancakes on top of my pork 'n' beans can. I would look up for his approval while manning my pancakes. He seemed distant and contemplative, like one who studies his next move. And there he shared with me, his ten-year-old daughter, his plan to end his life. He shared how the thought of losing my mother and the silence of home was just too much, and perhaps grabbing a knife from the drawer would end his consequent suffering.

I don't think my dad imagined a world where my mother would ever leave him. By the time my parents divorced, they had been together since high school, my father abusive the entire time. I think that just as my mother had grown into simply living with the abusive behavior of my father, my father had grown into his abuse and never imagined that my mother would leave. For him, it was yet another woman who would leave his side, much as his mother had done. Now he was the perpetrator of abuse and neglect, and above all, the proud owner of a deficit of love.

I wasn't there to hide the knives in his home. My young brain contemplated ways to prevent his possible plan and save the day, or at least my father. I didn't know how to process this information. In some ways, it felt familiar and almost expected behavior from him. By this age I had grown accustomed to my father being anything but stable. I wrestled with distinguishing between anger toward his possible cruel and familiar manipulation and empathy for his pain, and which emotion I would want to claim as my own. Truthfully, the acceptance of both of these sensations wouldn't come until much later. At that moment, all that I felt was my childlike fixation on making it okay. I wanted to make it okay for my parents, a weight that no child should ever have to carry. Eventually, he would bring me home to my grandmother's house, driving away.

You do not have to save the day.
You do not have to save the day.
You can save yourself and let go.

The next time I would see my father would be at my mother's funeral, almost twenty years later. After the service, I stood in front of the church's row of chairs, my legs edged against the seating, as mourners greeted our family, offering their condolences. I felt the need to smile as shock sent waves of disassociation through my body. I didn't want to just appear strong. I wanted to show how unbreakable I was. For better or worse, I cleaved to that smile plastered on my face, as if my stoicism in the face of my mother's death would make her proud. And for one reason or another, proud meant clinging to that simper as if it were the very thing that would save me from drowning in the sea of "Sorry for your losses" and "How are you's?"

I felt a hand grab my arm, pushing me toward one person and then another and then another. I felt seasick as I was transferred and passed between people until I landed in front of my two aunts. My father's sisters had not seen me since I was eight or nine years old. They embraced me and quickly propelled me closer to a tall, familiar figure. And there he was, my father, Greg.

My relationship with Greg had died moments after my mother packed our bags to leave many years prior. And because of this, seeing him after so many years was like witnessing a specter risen from the grave. I hadn't seen him since I was ten years old, and here I was approaching thirty. However, talking to him this time felt different from when I was a child. Although he stood well over six feet tall, he didn't seem as big as he did when I was a child.

Greg's breath smelled of hard liquor. His voice seemed like a voice without a home or occupancy. I had forgotten the sound of his voice. He and I looked awkwardly at each other like strangers reacquainted. Greg spoke. I listened, watching. This tower of a man who used to frighten me as a child now appeared childlike, sheepish almost. He talked fast and as if his words were in a race to escape his lips. I could tell that he had an ocean's worth of words that he wanted to say to me before the next person approached me and caused me to sail away once again and perhaps forever. He expressed his regret, saying "I'm sorry. And I love you." I wasn't sure if he was, like everyone else present that day, expressing his regret for the loss of my mother. Or if he was apologizing for the harm he'd committed, the death of my childhood, or perhaps contribution to my mother's demise.

As he continued his apologies, I saw him. Within this ghost of a man, I saw a little boy, not my father. I saw a little boy who grew up not feeling the touch of a loving hand from his mother. I saw a little boy afraid of me, and perhaps of my expected response to his past behavior and abuses. Standing there, I was no longer the child sitting with her father on the park bench. I was an adult and a mother, staring at a boy who had fumbled the opportunity of growing into not only his manhood but his personhood as well. I saw a person so emotionally stunted, fearful, and, most important, unaware of who he was. He was unaware of anything outside the moment. Unaware of the hurt caused by his hands. His presence overshadowed my mother, the woman he punched and kicked and performed a multitude of sins against, lying there in a coffin.

I never considered what I would do or say if I ever saw him face to face as an adult. However, at that moment, I remembered the stories that my mother shared with me about the abandonment and abuse he suffered as a kid. I saw his trauma and just how unhealed hurt passes down like oil, dripping onto those within its vicinity. I also imagined the act of not adorning my child with love, and the multitude of seeds of recovery one would need from that type of violence received. There before me at my mother's funeral was a boy, not a man, a hurt human, not a monster. And at that moment, the hatred that I had felt toward my father and the unforgiveness died that day also. My mother's funeral would be the last time I saw my father alive. He said "I love you," to which I said "I love you too."

It's okay to want to let go
It's okay to wrestle
Goodbye can also mean I love you.

DEATH AS THE BEGINNING

There are numerous ways that death presents in our lives. As mentioned, there is the physical death that occurs when we lose those who matter to us. There is also the death of things that we lose as we proceed onward and upward to our mountaintop. Just as my goal was to normalize grief in the previous chapters, I want you to normalize death and reframe it as perhaps the start of things instead of merely the end. I would like to reframe it simply as a letting go, a release.

When we think of death, many of us recall funerals. We are reminded of loss and the feeling of emptiness that death leaves behind. There are many forms, shapes, and variations of gray.

When we study our life cycles and the many iterations of ourselves and our becoming, we can observe that death precedes many new beginnings. For things to bloom, we must make space, allowing the rigid leaves beneath our feet to continue to grow rigid as the wind crisps them, crinkling them beneath our feet to die. When I saw my father for the first and, unbeknownst to me, the last time after my mother died, I felt anger, fear, and all of the emotions that one would imagine toward someone who had caused such harm. My feelings toward my father were resentment and helplessness, if the two could exist. I felt immense resentment toward my father as one of the many thieves of my childhood. With his words and violence, he robbed me of playtime and playing pretend, infecting my childhood with the need for hypervigilance and razor-sharp awareness of my surroundings. I was wise beyond my years because I had to be. After years of managing and trying my hand at keeping the two adults in my life safe by my childhood ritualistic practice of hiding knives so many years ago, I still could not prevent at least one of them from dying.

There's so little that the grown-ups tell you as a child, although, as children, what we perceive and take in overshadows our ability to actually process the weight of what we innately know. I, for one, knew that my father was unstable and that something was wrong. I knew that my father could not provide the security that I needed and craved as a child. I kenned the visceral feelings of fear and unpredictability that his very presence evoked when he walked into our home. And because of this, hatred was not the only feeling that I felt toward him, but also sadness. Sadness that in the park, he thought to tell his daughter his plans for suicide instead of a story of make-believe, dragons, and happily-ever-afters. My heart hurt for the little girl who had to sit there and listen, contemplating how she could be like the prince in the storybooks and save the day, hiding all the knives and sharp objects one by one.

Just as I was able to see nothing more than a tall boy standing before me at my mother's funeral, I was now able to perceive the death of my hatred and discontent toward my father as well. Greg lacked the capacity for the kind of love that children and many people need. He didn't know how to love himself. And when love is not known, held close to our bosom, it is impossible to share it with those around us, even if we genuinely wish to. My father lacked the tools to stand a chance against his demons, between undiagnosed mental illness and self-medicating. Back then, many people would throw out a term like "crazy," painting it across all who perhaps needed a good look at what was going on upstairs. The idea that somehow my father could show up for me in a fraction of the way that many parents show up for their children was the equivalent of asking a beggar for a hundred dollars. He couldn't give what he didn't have.

Unfortunately, many people grow up in homes with parents who could not love them from a healthy place. I want you to know that there is nothing that you could have done to make them love you more. And that there is nothing that you did to make the adults love you less than what you deserved. Many of our parents were not afforded the tools that we have now. And while this is not an excuse for continued harm, recognizing it can aid in our growing perspective and how we heal through past hurts and dysfunction. Some of our parents were oversized children with unhealed trauma and trigger responses doing their best.

The more I explored my thoughts around emotional death, I found that my mother was not exempt. There were many ways that I would have to allow our relationship's death and grieving process to take shape. For years, most of my anger would be aimed at my father, as he was the perpetrator of the abuse, not my mother. Like my sister and me, she was a victim. While my sister and I were there to see the abuse, my mother was the one whose face met the back of his hands. Witnessing this behavior leaves one feeling unprotected. It wasn't fair that, as a child, I had to see these things. Part of the reason I continued to see what I saw was twofold. My father was abusive and violent, and unfortunately, my mother stayed. I lived a large portion of my childhood in fear because of my parents' actions and lack thereof. My father's violence, and my mother's lingering within it.

Sitting with this reality felt like a betrayal of my mother. She was terrified of leaving. Perhaps the death of a relationship that she had known, no matter how violent and catastrophic, felt too hard a task to perform until it was not. I held on to my mother's blamelessness because accepting my mother's hand in the death of my girlhood was too hard an ask for me too. She was perfect.

She was strong. And in my mind, I wanted and needed her to stay that way. I didn't know then that she could be all of these things and her choices could also be culpable in the shit that I would have to work through. She didn't protect me from the shouts and fights that I heard at night. She didn't protect me from the uncle who molested me. And allowing the notion that my mother had no ownership in the stuff that I would have to sort through, no matter how inherently good a mother she was, did nothing for my healing. My mother tried, and she also failed. Both were true.

There are no perfect people,
as there is no perfect magic.

FUNGI, OUR TEACHER

One of my favorite features of nature to study is the mushroom. I've always been fascinated by how fungi develop, breaking down the dead things and then blooming nourishment and growth possibilities for the entire ecosystem. When an animal dies in the forest, its body begins to decompose and fungi break down the animal. The fungi feed on the dead organism. Once it has deteriorated, it becomes a part of the soil, becoming food for the surrounding plants and trees. Without death, there is no beginning. Without the wilting away and the slow decomposing of that which is no longer, there is no soil, no rich dark environment for nature to grow.

The same is true for us. Suppose we want to enjoy and welcome the nurturing of our environment. In that case, there must also be the work of allowing all that no longer supports our thriving to die. It's hard to let things go. It's hard to release certain relationships and our adherence to particular viewpoints. We begin to attach outlooks, relationships, thought patterns, and actions to who we are. We marry them, form a union, and even say till death do us part. What ideas have you married that no longer push your growth forward? Those things are hard to let die. But it would be in our best interest to do so. Also, I should note that some deaths are not instant. In some cases, there is a process of slow decomposition bit by bit. Both are okay.

Example: The breaking down and deterioration of beliefs about ourselves and others is a prominent example of such a slow burn and release. This kind of death doesn't come easy, nor is it painless. And I get it. Once we recognize it, we want it to die right away. The end of believing that we are undeserving of _____ is slow. The demise of hoping that _____ could have or would have been different is also a slow death. And trust me, I get it. Many of us would wish not to prolong the end of the things we want to release. We want the end of carrying such disappointment to come quickly so that we no longer feel the suffering. We don't want to feel it anymore. However, it takes what it takes. Death, the end, the release of what no longer grows us or aids in our healing, often is long work.

So, how do we thrive while grieving the end? We reimagine death not solely as the end of a thing, but also the beginning. The death of my resentment toward Greg birthed empathy and my ability to identify him as simply a hurt person who hurt people. The death of my refusal to acknowledge the unrecognized anger that I had toward my mother was the birth of my understanding that she did the best that she knew how. Sometimes it was enough, and sometimes it was not. Death is just another form of releasing and letting go. One of the many takeaways I gathered during my psychedelic trip was that we are all needing and sometimes desperately attempting to let go of something.

My attachment to anxiety, checking my surroundings, and hypervigilance I had been holding to myself, hands clutched. It wasn't until I began doing work and saw that my overly cautious nature was purely linked to my survival, not who I am, that I could let go of it. Sure, as I mentioned earlier in the book, the thing or the figure I was holding on to, which was hovering above me in space, looked like me. However, it was lifeless, a statue, purely a replica of who I was, only because I had become one with the survival tool, so much so that it resembled me. However, it was not me. It wasn't until I saw the lifelessness of what I was holding on to that I was able to detach from it and let it go. My point is, we are all attaching and holding on to the things that no longer serve us, sometimes struggling to let them go and release them. My parents' things were no different from mine or yours. My father's drug addiction was birthed out of his survival and coping through childhood trauma. My mother's stay in a violent marriage was birthed out of fear of leaving the familiar, even if it was rooted in chaos. All of it was hard to let go of and disengage from. My thing was no different from theirs or yours. It is not better or worse. Hard things are hard things, and releasing *is* hard. I say to folks that we are all experiencing our version of hard. We are all experiencing our own version of letting go. However, I'll tell you, as I tell myself: I (we) can let go.

My parents knew what they knew. And what they didn't know, they just didn't. They didn't realize that by not dealing with and healing their wounds, they would pass along those same wounds to their children, like a love letter of curses gifted to a friend, not an enemy. My father didn't mean to hurt me with his words, with his violence, just as my mother didn't mean to hurt me with her fear of leaving. My father didn't realize that by not putting to death his relationship with self-medicating, he would leave a daughter feeling the need to compete for the kind of allegiance he had to his drugs of choice. My mother didn't know that by not putting to death her relationship with my father sooner than later, her prolonging would leave a lasting effect on me not feeling safe enough, trusting enough, and afraid of any unknown threat. They didn't know.

KNOW YOUR ANGER

In this realization, something shifted. Despite the many ways my parents failed, despite their deficits, unknowns, and imperfections, I began to feel their love. I began to feel and know that they loved me—my parents were just two flawed people who came together trying their best to outlast the day.

My parents' flaws had nothing to do with me. They were two young adults coping as best they could. Why was knowing that I am loved and was loved important? Because it takes the motive of one's decisions away from the recipient. My father wasn't abusive because he didn't love me. He was abusive because he didn't know how to express his anger nonviolently. The love we express outwardly and speak of is bestowed upon us and within us.

So how do we thrive while accepting death? We must know and name our anger. You cannot heal what you do not know. One of my favorite quotes regarding anger is by the activist Gloria Steinem: "The truth will set you free, but first, it will piss you off!" There is a process to truth and how we metabolize its actualization. If we are going to sit with truth, we must sit with all of it, the ugly parts included, as most often those are the parts that free us. I only wanted to acknowledge the beautiful parts of my mother, not the parts that she perhaps lay blamable for in my continuance of childhood trauma. However, choosing to see and touch only my mother's "good parts" is not mending. It is not a holistic love. Refusing to acknowledge her human flaws is love in partiality. It's not whole. For me to continue to love her, I would have to see and accept the hurt caused by her hands as well.

As with any form of grief, there is the initial shock, denial, bargaining, and then unapologetic (yet often apologetic) anger. For years, I masked my rage regarding the traumatic events of childhood. When my mother found love and remarried when I was in middle school, I had a relatively happy adolescence afterward. I didn't think I had room or the right to be angry over my early childhood's more formative and developmental years. I now had a happy childhood ending. Ronald, my stepdad, had ridden up on his white horse, rescuing us all. How dare I feel anger?

Just as I had to mourn the death of my mother and even my father, I also had to mourn my childhood. I had to let die the asking and bargaining for me to change it somehow. Being a kid was traumatic. To mourn it, I had to first acknowledge it for what it was, burying it beneath the marigolds conducting its funeral procession. I had to grieve for the little girl who didn't feel safe. As part of my process, I wrote a letter to my childhood self, and I suggest the same for you, listing all the things you are allowing to die and release to the good earth. We may not be able to revisit those moments of trespass and violation. But we can kiss our wounds by offering ourselves precisely what we need to heal forward. There is something very healing about putting pen to paper and writing a letter to yourself. It is a unique way of processing. These are words that I've written to myself. I want you to consider them as your own as well:

Dear Brandi,

    I am so very sorry. I am sorry that you had to see so much as a little girl. And because of that had to dig your way out of feeling unsafe, unseen, and at times unloved. I am sorry that you had to keep the two people you loved as a child from killing each other or killing themselves. I am sorry that you had to find ways to manage the anxiety and, at times, depression of it all. I want you to know that it is not your fault. It is not your fault that you skim over the checklist of your mind to keep you protected. It is not your fault that you try your best to manage those around you, also keeping them safe, ensuring that you never cause hurt or harm. I am sorry that you have carried the weight of this around with you. I want you to know that you can release it. That I, adult Brandi, can take it from here. Your adult self is doing the work to unlearn the unhealthy parts that have silenced you and kept you frozen in fear. I want you to know that you no longer have to manage to feel protected. The only times that you need to show up are when joy is present and when you are living your wildest childhood dreams. Which, by the way—you are. You no longer have to manage, prepare, and build walls like pillow forts, soft, impractical, yet so dependent upon. We are no longer in danger and are safe. I promise not to silence you. Your words matter. Your safety matters. Your presence matters. However, I will be creating a bit of boundary and reassignments to your overall role within our current life moving forward. You are a part of me. You are the beautiful and protective parts. However, you can now drop that latter role and step into the joyful, beautiful, curious, and free parts. I know that it may take a bit of unlearning, but I've got you. We will do this together.

COMMUNAL GRIEF

I get asked a lot about how I show up for souls in grief. Perhaps you have a friend who has encountered loss and is experiencing a variant of death. I want to talk about the power of communal grief and why it's essential to our thriving. Death or suffering is not meant to be experienced alone but in the arms of the community. In chapter 9, I expressed the importance of reaching outward, accessing all of our resources when experiencing loss. However, we all know that many times we don't do this. Many who are knee-deep in pain don't want to be viewed as a burden. They don't want to be the extra thing for someone to think about or add to their list. So many, unfortunately, suffer in silence. This is where communal grief comes in.

When it comes to communal grief, we can learn from our mushroom friends and what is known as the mycelium network. This network is composed of the fungi's fibers reaching deep beneath the ground's surface. These weblike fibers expand and interlock, touching hands like many of us who yearn for connection when contact seems scarce. The mycelium network extends miles and miles beneath the forest floor. What's so important about this internet-like network is that it acts as a means of communication between plants and trees. Tall redwoods use this network to communicate with other redwoods and plant species to meet their needs or to ward away danger. For example, a tree that may lack nutrients and is sick will communicate using this mycelium network to borrow nutrients from other trees.

If nature has this dance of giving and taking, bartering between acceptance and goodbyes, so should we as humans. When we see those within our mycelium network in grief experiencing loss, this is the time to show up for them as well, gifting the life-giving sap and nutrients from our soil. This showing up can look like dropping off a meal at their doorstep. If they want to talk, it may just be listening. Sometimes it is sitting in silence. Showing up for those experiencing death and allowing others to show up for us is a replicated act of nature. Knowing and owning that we are not a burden when we call on and lean into our mycelium network for support is how we can and should be.

When supporting each other through loss, I usually suggest asking direct questions that don't require the person in grief to think. Avoid questions like "Is there anything you need?" Because many people don't know what they need during grief, unfortunately. I usually ask direct questions like "Have you eaten today? May I buy you lunch?" "Are you drinking water?" Or I send a care package. These are ways to be there for those who have suffered a loss and are healing their wound.

How does one create a mycelium network? Your network can contain just a few people within your village. A support network is not about numbers but instead intentional support. This group of people is a lifeline of constant communication. I suggest each person take turns checking in, dropping by, and showing up for the person who needs support.

To thrive while experiencing loss, we open ourselves. It is expected to want to go back, taste, and touch our way back to what was lost. It's okay to want to reason and for us to feel the push and pull of bargaining and pleading to go back to the old. Trust me. I've played this game of tug-of-war as well. I've had one foot in the present while dipping my toe in the anguish for what was lost. How I got over? You don't. There is no set arrival. However, there is an adventure. There is a journey. To thrive while experiencing loss is not about making peace, but about making the decision to let the dying die, allowing it to be as it is without additives. If it doesn't grow, we can let go.

- What are you releasing? What does the end look like?
- Identify your mycelium network.
- Write a letter to all that you are releasing.

CHAPTER ELEVEN

Surviving a Seasonal Shift

And there she was in her boat and lost at sea.

She didn't mean to find herself there, yet there she was, nestled between waves and miles away from shore, transfixed between the sun that kissed the waters and complete darkness at the very bottom of the ocean's floor. There she was in her small boat, surrounded by what seemed to be endless nothingness, alone. Beneath her were bright fish, marine life that she had both caught and was familiar with as a fisherwoman on the island. However, knowledgeable as she was about the sea, fear, wonder, and everything below the water's surface existed. Sure, she had ventured out into the deep before. However, she had never found herself lost at sea, with the threat of being buried beneath its waves.

She had intended to set out on an adventure. She'd heard tales of an ancient mountain that bloomed with all sorts of flowers and mushrooms, plants that could heal a person and produce wealth through magic. And instead, somehow, here she was at the will of the sea, its waves, and perhaps the sea monsters below, with nothing but a meager meal meant for a day and an extraordinary tapestry knitted together by mothers, grandmothers, great-aunts, and aunties for moments like this.

She yelled to the sky. How was it possible that after having prepared as much as she had for this mountaintop experience, she'd encountered such a blow? Had she missed something? Rain began to fall from the sky. The lightning crashed, and the thunder rumbled. The ship rocked and swayed violently against the waves as she attempted to tame the storm around her. The forceful winds caused the boat's sail to break. Without the sail, there was no hope for the girl or the ship to survive such turbulence. So she quickly grabbed the tapestry from her bag, hoping to climb to the top of the mast and attach it. She hoped that the tapestry would be strong enough to allow her to gain some control of the boat. However, it was all too strong for her between the lawless tides and the unpredictable storm. And so she surrendered to it. She'd come so far because of the waves of the ocean. Perhaps they would show compassion and continue to carry her forward? She closed her eyes, remembering the many ways by which these same waves had allowed her to catch fish, providing for her family. Perhaps her submission to and trust of the storm's process was the offering she could bestow in reciprocity to the sea? The sea was there to carry her, not bury her. She closed her eyes once again. And just like that, it was over.

The young fisherwoman seemed to finally reach her destination. However, she had a bridge to cross, and then she could begin the hike up to her mountain. The bridge was flimsy and worn. Each step, no matter how unfamiliar, felt terrifying. This high and rickety bridge connected the girl from sea to land, from complete despair and loss to her mastery. The earsplitting fear that met her in the ocean seemed to follow her here. However, as she climbed closer and closer to the top, she felt a sense of promise emerge. She saw it. She had survived all manner of turmoil, the unsettled nature of the sea, hunger, and the pathway to the mountaintop. She reached her mountain. However, there were no treasures or healing plants but an inscription covered in moss. It read, "You are here." The fisherwoman read the words, reflecting on her journey and the meaning of it all. Being here was the reward of survival, and that in itself was the treasure pursued.

Grief is often congested with our obsession with the happily-ever-after and our need for resolve, when there may never be such. It is filled with either-or, black and white, and a desire for precise measurement and exactitude, when really grief is like the smell of smoke, lingering until it is no longer, marrying itself at some point to us all. When there is loss, there is grief. When there is abundance, there is also grief. Life is a not-so-seamless dance between the two: contentment and sorrow intertwined.

When we think of grief and loss, we only consider them when death is present. However, I believe that we all grieve in some manner or another after manifesting or birthing our dreams. It's not uncommon that after receiving the call for the dream career or hearing the good news that you've been hoping for, one may experience feelings of grief for all that was lost in the process of arriving at a place called here. One may ask why I would include postpartum (or after manifesting) experience in the section on grief and loss, primarily when most people associate loss with death? For many, death is the antithesis of birth. However, as a birth guide, we know the risk of going into childbirth. We also know the close association between birth and death. For anything to be born, something must die. After birthing a baby, one delivers the placenta, only for this once life-sustaining organ to

eventually begin its new mission of decomposition.

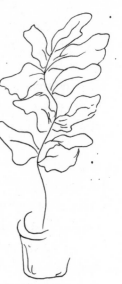

And yes, the grief that occurs post-birth
does include you even if you are not a parent. When I reference the term "post-birth"
or "postpartum," I am referencing physical
birth as well as the intuitive manifestation
of our deepest desires and dreams, both
spoken and unspoken. I am referencing
what we must do to thrive after birthing the
things whispered in the dead of night.

DORMANCY IN GRIEF

I will start by saying that survival paired with repose is one of the
keys to thriving during a season of grief. When one is in the thick
of grief, "doing nothing" is everything. I know, this is a book
about thriving. Often when we hear the word "thriving," we in-
ternalize it as a resolute call to action and a laundry list of feelings to ignore and conquer. However, we must first make it to
and through another day to thrive. I want you to know that the
simple yet impactful act of showing up for yourself (however
that presents from day to day) is worthy of celebration and acknowledgment. Your current movement is both large and significant, no matter how small it may feel. Where do you start?
You likely already have with dormancy.

Dormancy is a thriving strategy employed by our plant friends
when encountering a change in temperature, seasonal or otherwise. During this time, plants will halt all manner of growth,
bearing fruit, and productivity to conserve energy for the unknown and challenging road ahead. While it is dormant, you will
not find your favorite fern sprouting new leaves. It is too busy

trying its best to persevere by simply doing what seems to be in its best interest of growth, which is in this case doing nothing (I know, this can be hard for us doers).

The same is true for trees, who recognize that while they can't control the uncertainty of the weather, they can control their response to it. In the case of cold weather shifts, many trees will opt to slow down their growth cycle, go into a type of hibernation, and shed their leaves, as keeping them requires quite a bit of energy, which they can't afford to exhaust. While dormant, many trees will slow down their nutrient intake and metabolism to heighten their chances of survival.

These wise trees and your favorite houseplant know that they must first survive to thrive. Within this chess-like strategy, they wait until favorable conditions for growth, output, and usual intake to begin. Nature knows that there is no rushing or time stamp on navigating during dormancy, knowing that this is but a season. Sometimes life puts us in a place of dormancy without our even choosing, but you notice that you stop and need to simply survive the day-to-day before trying to accomplish anything. To thrive during the season of grief, dormancy is essential.

Janet, my fiddle fig, has taught me the most about dormancy. Now, Janet is one bad mutha. I purchased her many years ago when she was only about two feet tall. I was warned that she more than likely wouldn't survive well, as these types of plants were super inconsistent, and any form of disruption could send her reeling. I get it. This tenderoni plant was tender. However, I not only kept Janet alive well past what was expected by the shopkeeper, but Janet grew to be over ten feet tall, touching our living room ceiling. She arched over the west-facing window as she allowed the sunset to play a game of peek-a-boo through the separation of her leaves. There would be seasons where I would notice new branch after new branch budding and producing fresh leaves, almost as if she knew that everyone had counted her as the underdog. Janet wanted to prove us wrong. Janet was strong and wanted us to know it.

One day, as I was watering her, I noticed that I hadn't seen as many new leaves as I did before. I hadn't seen any for quite some time. It was as if she had gone through a cycle of growing and growing and blooming and more blooming, and then she stopped. One would think that perhaps she was dying? She didn't look like it. She had everything that she needed. However, it seemed nature had brought her growing to a complete stop. After researching, I realized that she was going through a dormancy phase. After all, the weather had shifted to colder temperatures. So Janet shifted as well. She rested and did not produce the lush green leaves that she seemed to grow so effortlessly before her dormancy.

I noticed that her absorption would take much longer when I watered her, as she even slowed her nutrient intake. However, let me tell you, Janet was unbothered by my expectations or frustrations with her. She proceeded with life as if my expectations had nothing to do with her and all to do with me. I'm not sure how long this phase lasted, but I am fully aware of when it seemed to end.

Janet left me no choice but to go along at her pace. I realized that I needed to play her game her way in order to support her. So, instead of watering her as frequently as I did in the hotter summer months, I would wait until she asked for water. After wetting her, I decided to rotate her. It is recommended to turn your plant 180 degrees every so often to allow ample sunlight on all the leaves, allowing them all a place in the sun. As I was rotating her, I noticed something. On the side that had been hidden away, as if in mourning, it sprouted a new three-foot branch of fresh leaves. The brand-new addition bashfully made its debut to the sun. Because of Janet's dormancy phase, she had not only made it through and survived but had also thrived, producing bountiful new fronds.

When navigating grief post-birth, think of Janet. One thing is for sure, and two things are for certain: Change is the only guarantee post-birth. Birthing a big move? You are presented with all the twists and turns of change that relocating offers. You finally birth your childhood dream of writing a book, and just around the bend, change calls for a redistribution of time and availability. Postpartum and change go together like peanut butter and jelly. And if we are wise, getting our loaf of bread ready is beneficial.

And so what do we do after experiencing such a monumental moment as birth? If we are honest, many of us do more. We ride the momentum, sometimes hoping and often in fear of the train slowing down a bit. However, in these moments, we must rest, catch our breath, and reflect on what we were able to pull off: birth. Dormancy plays a considerable part in our post-birth survival and thriving. Knowing when to cease production and the slowing down of intake and output is indispensable during this process.

While working as a birth and postpartum guide, I noticed that new parents often feel the need to produce results despite the magnificent task their bodies have just performed. They'd feel compelled to send off emails, answer phone calls, or demand that their bodies and minds snap back into what was before their birthing experience. Many who were used to being there for others struggled with allowing their community's love and support to show up for them. Many struggled with being still and knowing that their present state, leaky chests, aching body, and sleep-deprived best were all good and, most important, enough. I would affirm with them that post-birth is a time to conserve every ounce of energy to simply survive the new season you are in. Now is not the time to push through for those who have given birth. Nor is it the time to compare what others can accomplish while nurturing their dream to our personal journey. It is time to ask for support and slow your intake. It is time to be still and heal, allowing our bones to fuse back to their origin as they come home to themselves. And much like Janet, on the other side of surviving, you, too, will see a new branch springing forth.

Grief After Birth

In my experience, I've found that many postpartum parents must go through a mourning period. Mourning the person they once were and the life they once possessed. There's a mourning period for comfortable and accessible sleep, perhaps once obtained. I want to grant you all permission to grieve for everything that you may have lost along the way to your mountain. I want you to know that it's okay to miss and long for the imperative and what now seems trivial. You *can* feel both blissed out and buried alive. The "and" is where your growth happens, and I believe it is uniquely tied to our liberation. It unshackles us from unrealistic expectations and obligations of what we "should" or "should not" be feeling, connecting us to our humanness. It releases us from choosing a team (for example, Team Bliss or Team Buried Alive?). We can be both. Our friend "and" shows up in dazed yet overjoyed late nights. And I believe if we embrace it, "and" can carry us from seasons of productivity to seasons of fruition *and* after what may present as stagnation.

THE BRIDGE OF "AND"

So how do we thrive when feeling both blissed out and buried alive? We must build and travel (like the fisherwoman) our own bridge between grief and contentment. The bridge is our "and." We can be both excited *and* overwhelmed. Enamored with bliss *and* buried beneath it. I get it. Crossing that bridge is scary, as it can feel as if acknowledging our humanity subtracts from the celebration presented. It almost feels sacrilegious and ungrateful to ask ourselves to choose between the two emotions, when really there doesn't have to be a choice. Again, you can be both. There is room for happiness within the grief and the grief within the joy. I would hear from sleep-deprived parents the words "I'm so exhausted," with a quick follow-up of "But I love them [their new baby] so much." As if admitting their need for sleep (which is a human necessity) excluded the validity of their love. I hear "I have no time to get things done, and I am overwhelmed" with the follow-up "But I'm so grateful for this new relationship, opportunity, or adventure." Almost as if one truth cancels out the other, when it does not.

I believe that many people don't know that the bridge of "and" exists and that there is allowance to traverse it, connecting contraindicative emotions as different as land and sea. Sometimes, our conjoined feelings couldn't look more dissimilar. It can be scary, as acknowledging both feelings requires our exploration of those emotions and the perhaps long and shaky walk forward. Why is it terrifying? It is unfamiliar. Putting one foot of curiosity in front of the other, acknowledging that this step feels exciting, and then the next one feels uncertain, and then the next feels like hope, and then despair. And each step feels true based on where you are on the bridge of life. However, we must allow the bridge to carry us through to the other side.

So how? How do we not only cross the bridge of "and" but accept it as a beneficial tool to get from where we currently are to the other side?

1. **We cease the war.** We've all been there. Both sentiments fight for the light of day. We believe we must not only choose but also suppress the emotion we deem unworthy of being seen. How dare we voice when we are confounded by our new dream career? Wide-eyed excitement should only be present, right? Friends, not at all. We traverse our bridge of "AND" by acknowledging that both feelings are worthy of being witnessed by us.

2. **We bury our emotions alive.** Similar to what we resist persists, what we bury and sow into the earth also grows. When stuck on the bridge of "and," try this visual practice: First, excavate the suppressed and "unwanted" emotion. I encourage you to visualize yourself holding the avoided emotion in one hand. Try putting an image or face to the feeling you are holding. What is the cause of this feeling? Where is it blooming from? (Examples: I am overwhelmed because _____. I feel envious of my friend's new _____ because _____.) I heard a wise woman say no emotion is negative. Only our thinking makes it so. When we physically hold the unwanted within our hand with exploration and curiosity, we can show tenderness toward it.

3. **Once you have held the negative, visualize holding the "feel-good emotion."** Do you feel full when you think of this emotion? Perhaps you feel gratitude? Now imagine

yourself holding both feelings within the palms of your hands. Visualize neither emotion carrying more or less weight than the other unless you put it there.

4. **We cross the bridge of "and,"** knowing that our emotions are neither good nor bad, but instead always revealing what we need more of or perhaps what we can do without. Listen closely.

We thrive during our post-birth stage by accessing our surrounding resources for thriving. In the parable, the fisherwoman sacrifices her tapestry. She uses its remains as a sail to get her beyond the ocean. During the storm, she makes the difficult decision to offer up the tapestry that the maternal figures in her life knitted and sewed together. Her last sail was damaged in the storm, and without tying the fragmented tapestry to the mast, risking its destruction, she would have continued to be in a ship without a sail isolated in the ocean. The young girl tapped into her infinite wisdom to know that the sea was far too wide a beast for her to conquer on her own, so she used her resources to allow the tapestry to become her sail so she could navigate the waters safely.

Much like the ocean, grief, too, is a vast beast. Many of us feel like the young girl in the sea without a sail, sitting in deep isolation, alone. There is no one and nothing in sight for miles. Just ocean separating you from everyone else. Grief is not meant to be experienced alone but instead felt in the company of community. Let's explore the benefit of communal grief and its importance. I want you to know that it's okay to use all of the resources available for your survival, tapping into the sacred tapestries available on your boat. You do not have to go about this alone.

Know Your Resources

Whether you are on the mountaintop or the ocean, the grief that surrounds you can be both palpable and turbulent. Although on land, many people can still feel the isolation of mountaintop success, reminiscent of the sea. When you feel isolated, this is the time to lean into those around us as a resource.

After birthing Jupiter, we had many visitors dropping by and bringing food. Some would volunteer to take the other kids to school. Some would sit with Jupiter, rocking him as I finally found time to take a much-needed shower. Between the aforementioned triple feedings and pumping and utter exhaustion, allowing people to come in and love on our family was our saving grace. This communal coming together was my resource for survival. Jupiter's birth was so very different from my first post-birth experience. I was in my mid-thirties as opposed to my early twenties. By this time, I no longer felt compelled to demonstrate how strong I was by my ability to fold my underwear or continue life as usual. If my mother-in-law had been alive then, I would have allowed her to be everything she wanted to be in the space without the intimidation of fear or not measuring up to the expectations in my head and society. By the time I had Jupiter, I had embraced that much like labor, I would now have to find and embrace my transition between my former life and the present.

Adaptation

There is another component to using our surrounding resources for our thriving, which is **adaptation**. We can take a lesson from our underwater plants, such as phytoplankton, seagrass, and kelp, all of which have not only adapted to water life but use their environment to thrive. These plants absorb nutrients from the water, the very thing that could very well drown them. Because a soil bed is not present in the ocean, they attach their roots to rocks, anchoring themselves to their sturdiness so that they won't just float away with the tide. They use the water to support them and keep them afloat. When we study seagrass, which can be found at the bottom of the ocean floor, this plant gathers its energy from the very minimal amount of sunlight provided. Because of that, it has adapted to slow growth patterns, conserving its energy. When **experiencing post-birth grieving, identify your rocks**. To what can you attach yourself to keep you rooted when you could otherwise float away with the tide? What resource acts as an anchor in your environment within the uncertainty of new schedules, people, and external factors?

The other lesson we can gather from the sacrifice of the tapestry is that in reaching our mountain, **it's okay to grieve for the things lost along the way**. The young girl must mourn her tapestry on her way to her mountain, even though it was her only choice for survival. Sure, she made it to the top of the hill, but she lost her tapestry along the way.

Often in birth, many will say, "Well, at least you had a healthy baby." People may say this after a traumatic birth. They will also say, "Well, at least you know that you can get pregnant again." Well-meaning people will say this after hearing about a miscarriage. Others may say there's no need for tears over that one business that didn't quite work out as hoped. At least you learned what not to do. "There's always that other business idea you had." You may even hear that birthing that new startup has never been done before, and perhaps the loss outweighs the potential gain. So move on sans grief. Friends, family, colleagues, although their intent is to be helpful, sometimes forget that there is still mourning to do, as there is still a loss that has taken place. I have had the privilege of receiving great opportunities. However, my mother would be something (someone) that I have lost along the way. I cannot call her and share the good news with her. She is no longer here to celebrate with me. Therefore, every time something good happens, I must also grieve that I cannot share it with my mother. You may have stumbled upon an opportunity. But with the opportunity comes long hours or perhaps temporarily missing experiences that you may have otherwise had time to enjoy. It would be beneficial if you grieve or at least acknowledge the perhaps temporary loss of those things enjoyed previously. Grief does not make you a bad person. Nor does its existence express your lack of contentment or gratitude. Acknowledging the big and small things lost is our way of honoring what was exceptional and our appreciation for its permanence in our lives. Our lost (and sometimes reclaimed) tapestries allow the wind to enter our sails, carrying us to our destination.

After birthing Jedi, my middle son, I remember feeling lost and abandoned in the ocean. Jedi was both the pregnancy and birth that I had hoped for. We were finally here after experiencing a miscarriage. Before this point, I had paid my wages in tears, begging and pleading for the previous pregnancy to stay. Before miscarrying, I would imagine a daughter with braids, cornrowed with no rhyme or reason. Or perhaps a son with a small gap between his front teeth like his father's. All of this would go away the moment I began to bleed. Naturally, I would try to reason with my womb to keep the baby within it, and instead, weeks later, my body would decide to let it all go. I couldn't look at the small piece of flesh that came out of my body. I felt it as it exited. And although I would like to say that I "bravely" held the tiny being within my hands, I did not and could not. I was in the bathroom on the toilet when it happened. By this time, there was no wailing left, as I had yelled what felt like guttural lament at the heavens for the past three weeks as I bled while on bed rest. I had nothing left to give and no penance left to pay for this sorrow and wound. Jon would come and gather it, putting it in safekeeping and then eventually casting it away, as one hopes to do with grief itself.

Although this miscarriage would be the catalyst for the work I needed to do, while I was steeped in it, there was no pathway through in sight. Miscarriage hollowed me as it emptied the birth from my womb. It's tough to come so close and finally touch what one has hoped for, only for it to leave your body without consent or say. A considerable part of humaning is experiencing the deep lament of "almost," bleeding and staining through what might have been. As children, we hear "Try again" as we attempt and fall and attempt again. And although I would go on to become pregnant again and eventually birth, the miscarriage experienced didn't disappear simply because of birth. And the same is so for you. Sometimes, miscarriage happens. You almost get the promotion, the partnership, the hoped-for plan, and then miscarriage happens. How do we move through, honoring our loss, even when on the other side?

1. Like the restless waves tossing our boat to and fro, we give our loss permission to shake and rock us. Our surrender is an offering to the sea and what was lost to it.
2. We yield to grief's sensations and the reminder that this loss enveloped our bellies once upon a time, filling us with light and hope.
3. We carry what we lost along the way with us. You do not have to leave your losses behind, nor do you have to simply get over them before moving forward.

4. Resolve and healing are not the same. Resolve or "getting over it" may never come, although healing will (if we allow it).

When I finally gave birth to Jedi, I felt joy like nothing else. Although there would be many things that I would change in the subsequent delivery, this particular birth experience felt like it was on my terms. However, the after-birth experience was an entirely different one. This birth was harrowing. I gave birth to Jedi almost forty-eight hours after my water broke. And because of this, like many babies who no longer have the protection of amniotic fluid and its sac after twenty-four hours, Jedi encountered the risk of developing an infection or newborn sepsis. As a result, Jedi and our family spent ten days in the NICU.

The pediatrician on call came into our postpartum hospital room. Expressionless vagueness filled her words. She mentioned something or another about Jedi needing to be taken into the NICU to be further evaluated because of his initial numbers from his newborn blood test, and then something about a spinal tap to rule out meningitis. That was it. I asked, "Do you know what's wrong? Is there something wrong?" They gave no clear answers. They shared with me all of the possible outcomes if they *didn't* perform a spinal tap if something were amiss. I stood there clutching my baby, shaking and confused. I was already experiencing postpartum fog, where absolutely nothing makes sense. It was too much for my brain at that moment to comprehend. I opened my arms reluctantly, giving my baby to the NICU nurse. I didn't know what else to do beyond what seemed to be already set in motion. I felt out of control, afraid, and wholly detached from the walls surrounding me. And just like that, they whisked my new baby away, along with the ecstasy experienced just moments before.

The hospital social worker whispered to Jon, "Let's keep an eye out for postpartum depression." How else did this woman expect me to respond to this kind of news? I believe hearing that their baby needed a spinal tap to rule out an infectious disease and the possibility of brain damage would send anyone into an emotional tailspin.

As I roamed the corridors of the NICU, the halls smelled of cleaning solutions and hand sanitizer. The NICU was down the hall, around the corner, and through two locked doubled doors. The NICU nursery's white walls were blinding, summoning a sense of perfection within the unexplained, and for some, unfortunate. What had been an empowering experience quickly turned into one of fear and the unfamiliar. The doctors and nurses made their morning rounds, reading from their clipboards. Numbers and stats are all that I heard and yet didn't understand. I just listened through the postpartum haze for some indication that Jedi was okay.

He underwent the spinal tap, and they could rule out meningitis. However, his bilirubin levels, levels that indicated signs of jaundice, were high, so this was also a factor beyond his initial infection. Jedi would lie in his light-filled incubator, which resembled a baby spaceship straight out of your favorite sci-fi movie. I left his side only to pump and when the NICU nurses would beg me to get some sleep. I wanted to be close to him, wrapped up in a blanket lying in our bed at home together. I ached for the vision that I had hoped for and read about. I had read all the books, taken all the birthing classes. I prepared for everything except this. And by this, I mean the grief that would have to settle like dust after birthing.

I felt isolated in my post-birth grief. I didn't want to be here in the NICU, mourning the loss of my fairytale post-birth. I would make my hourly walk from my hospital bed to the NICU between my strictly scheduled pumping sessions, sashaying in my salmon-colored slip-proof hospital socks to Jedi's side, to stare at him and hold him close. There were so many wires in his NICU makeshift crib. There were wires to monitor his blood pressure, oxygen levels, and heartbeat, accompanied by a little red cuff on his tiny foot to monitor his temperature. This kid was only days old and had experienced a spinal tap. I figured this was the worst thing ever to happen at that moment, or he was going to be badass. Only God would know.

I was one of the lucky ones. Many of the parents in the NICU were there for what seemed like no end in sight. Some of their babies received life-altering news, the kind that shakes you to your core, forever changing their stories and what they hoped and envisioned their children's lives to be. These parents seemed to have a far greater grieving process than me. One by one, I would see them be so very strong after hearing what I could only imagine being their worst nightmare. Some would break down, while others would breathe between the sobs, allowing their bodies to melt and become one with the chair beneath them. The NICU was filled with ambiguity and imperceptible news, hard for anyone to hold and claim as their own. So many here came to the hospital hoping to reach their mountain, only to land in this room, sacrificing so very much to grab hold of their glimmering moment of promised rapture.

We returned home from the hospital on what seemed to be one of the hottest days of that summer. Los Angeles was experiencing one of its many August heat waves. We arrived home to a heat-ravaged apartment. Jedi was nestled to my chest, wrapped and swaddled close. I stripped us both naked, allowing the skin-to-skin contact that I'd yearned for in the NICU. I remember plopping down on the sofa, thinking about how our birth, what seemed to be my mountain, had been this magical experience and how my post-birth left its own set of circumstances to be mourned. My postpartum experience was traumatic—my baby being in the NICU was also traumatic. I had to grieve the post-birth experience that I had envisioned. My grieving process resembled the resolution that "My birth experience was wonderful, *and* the beginning of my postpartum experience was trash." Trust me. I also tried to make only lemonade out of the bitter lemons handed to me. I did the very thing I'm recommending that you don't do. I reasoned and counted my blessings one by one. However, I found that by not mourning the lost parts, I erased their existence and my experience. And if I erase my experience, I run the risk of erasing perhaps valuable aspects of my tapestry, reclaimed for you and anyone that has found themselves confined between waves and alone at sea.

Grief as a Compass

We thrive during grief by knowing where we are. Here. Similar to the young fisherwoman who finally arrives at the top of the mountain in search of treasure, only to find a tablet reminding her of where she is—well, that is the treasure. Knowing where your feet are is a gift and can serve as an internal GPS. Grief can create a sense of disassociation, separating the head from the heart and even the present. For those of us who have lost loved ones, if we close our eyes, we can time-jump right back to their bedside, holding their hands and saying our goodbyes. We can remember what the room smelled of and how their hands felt intertwined with ours. And then, when we open our eyes, our body is here in the present.

The abundance is knowing where we are in the world, despite our emotions and the external stimuli and triggers. It grounds us in our reality so that we can continue to progress and grow. An exercise that my dear friend Christina, who had experienced their own measure of grief, shared was the practice of reminding yourself where you are by looking down at your feet. Sit down on a chair and look at your feet. Whisper to yourself, "I am here. My feet are here. My feet are on the ground. The ground supports me. It is here to support me." When we experience moments of a mountaintop or post-birth grief, we must remind ourselves where we are and just how much we encountered and experienced and endured to be, *here*. The locating, in this case, is both a practice of grounding and a celebration. You are *here, and* you are *here*!

Grief is hard work and heart work. As mentioned, it is like the smell of smoke, marrying itself to all who experience this thing called life. However, like the smoke of sage or copal that caresses the walls of cathedrals, it leaves a fragrance of tenderness and connection with human existence. Although it may feel as if we are at sea, we are never entirely alone. Under the young fisherwoman's feet, deep beneath the ocean's surface, were millions of plants just like her, persisting, adapting, anchoring themselves to survive another day so that they, too, could thrive.

- **Identify your tapestry.** Identify the resources that can act as a sail when lost at sea and/or experiencing stormy weather.
- **Recognize your rocks.** To what can you attach your roots to stay grounded?
- **Identify possible dormancy within your grief.** Journal ways you can implement gentleness (for example, slower intake and output, or conservation of energy) within your grief process.

PART FOUR

. . . .

Thriving While Othered

Dinah, the Philodendron Selluom

The Philodendron, she reaches over and under her plant friends, unashamed, reclaiming her space.

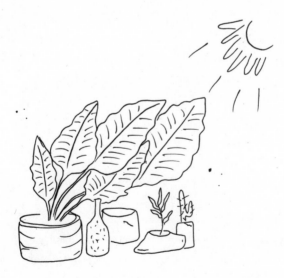

CHAPTER TWELVE

Othered and Thriving

My cousins and I would spend the hot, humid days playing outside in the sprinklers during the summer, as there was no such thing for us as summer camp. After all, we had each other's company. We would eat ice with food coloring and syrup out of Styrofoam cups, after which our tongues would be bright red or some shade of radioactive blue-green. We would ride our bicycles up and down the steep hill adjacent to my grandmother's home. I remember barreling down the hill adjacent to my grandmother's home and crashing full speed into a fence. In no time, I was up and riding my bicycle, making my way back up that same steep hill.

The sweltering summer days would turn into equally hot and humid summer nights of us kids running around, catching lightning bugs, and staying up way past our bedtime. Our hair would sweat out and dismantle any form of taming of our wild child tresses. Beads of sweat would fall across my cousins' brow. I wanted to sweat like them. The amount of sweat you had to wipe away was proof of how much fun you were experiencing as a child. Unfortunately, my evidence of enjoyment would only materialize on my back.

During the day, my cousins and I would venture into town. Now and then, we would run into another kid or adult, someone who may not have known our family in its entirety. These intrusive strangers would automatically assume that I was a family friend and not one of the cousins. Some of the strangers would search our faces, looking for any similarities. I could see their eyes tracing and comparing our noses and eyes. Perhaps they will see it in our mouth? Our smiles and high cheekbones were kind of similar. I was rooting for them to see it. If they saw our similarities, that would mean that I belonged, a desire and need we all possess. We want to *belong* to those we call kin and those who encircle our daily lives. I wasn't unique in this hope. I'm sure that you, too, despite your individual differences, would pray on bended knees that these differences wouldn't stand in the way of your being seen as a part of the group but instead would be swallowed up in full support and acceptance. Maybe you imagined a world where these differences weren't a part of your story, and perhaps they would disappear altogether. So much so that if being "different" were the price to pay in exchange for belonging, you would gladly consider it an option. As a child, I imagined myself with lighter skin like my cousins and like their mothers. Perhaps you also imagined a different existence in the spirit of belonging?

Some strangers would assume that two-thirds of our group were related, leaving me as the outsider. I could hear their assumption in their body language. They would address my lighter-skinned cousins, not me. Or they would say to my lighter-skinned relative, "so this is your cousin?" and exclude me altogether. I preferred the latter. It made it less awkward, as I was uncomfortable enough. I was darker. Was this what the poet Langston

Hughes meant when he said that he is the darker brother? I re-member, at that moment, feeling different. Other. I would search my cousins' faces for similar features. My nose was differ-ent, resembling my father's long and broad nose. My eyes and skin color were both different. I didn't see myself in my cousins or on television. Back then, there was no Lupita Nyong'o or Viola Davis. There for darn sure wasn't a First Lady Michelle Obama. There were only women who resembled Clair Huxtable, Lisa from *Coming to America,* or Grace Jones. For the record, *now* I adore Grace Jones and what she stood for. However, a five-year-old kid singing, let alone watching Ms. Jones perform "Pull Up to My Bumper" wasn't necessarily age-appropriate. All of this spoke volumes to little girls with dark skin like mine. It expressed the idea "You are not enough." Or at least not enough to be fully seen. While I don't remember a moment in which I was unaware of my Blackness, I remember every moment in which I was made to feel that I was "other." This moment of ex-clusion was one of those moments. Well, this moment, and school picture day.

Like most children, I looked forward to picture day. I loved playing dress-up. This day was another excuse to wear my Sun-day best and get my hair done. I wore a blue and white seer-sucker dress with ruffled sleeves and thick white tights that I'd change out of as soon as the photographer took my picture. My mother and I stayed up late doing hair, meaning that my mother pushed back my bedtime. I remember her washing and blowing my hair dry and then using a hot comb to make it straight. See-ing the hot comb on the stove was an announcement in and of itself that our sacred ceremony was about to take place. The crackling sound of grease meeting comb and then meeting hair is a sound that most Black girls will never forget. The hissing of teeth sucking together as my mother accidentally burned the nape of my neck and ears. In my head, I'd unleash a string of cuss words that my mother would never hear. Picture day was the one day of the year that my mother allowed me to wear my hair down. I still remember the smell of the hot iron on top of the stove. It smelled of burnt hair and Blue Magic. My mother dipped her caramel-colored pointer finger into the grease and spread it onto a sectioned part of my hair. The hot comb sizzled as she combed it through.

My mother didn't know it then, but she was introducing me to a sense of ritual and connection. Although I was surrounded by many who didn't look like me and had no clue about our clandestine nighttime routine, this time was ours. And at that moment, it connected me to something greater, more profound, and far more comprehensive than the othering I was experiencing daily. This rebellious act of simply taking care, as rowdy as the unruly hair on my head, reminded me of my belonging to a greater community. This is what ritual does when we feel othered. Ritual allows us to soak the harms of othering in a healing balm of kinship. It quiets the voice that says "Because you are _____, you are not worthy of life, liberty, or the pursuit of joy." So tell me something. What is it that you connect to while experiencing feelings of being othered? What tethers you to those within your current community or those who came before, who fought the good fight so that you can live the life they dreamed of making manifest?

I grew up in the '80s, an epoch when Saturday morning cartoons, cereal, and the Jheri curl were an absolute thing. My aunts had wide hips and broad noses. My uncles were black as midnight, or as some would say, blue-black. My mother was the color of honey; my father was dark bitter chocolate. My cousins on my mother's side all had lighter skin. My skin was dark like my father's.

This skin was my existence. During class, I would sit next to a girl with shoulder-grazing pigtails. Her hair was silky and straight and smelled of Pert Plus. My hair didn't smell or look like hers or anyone else's in my class. Instead, my hair smelled of pink setting lotion. My mother and I would always find ourselves running late to school. In the car, my mother would quickly slather on this Pepto Bismol–colored magical elixir, setting my bangs onto a gigantic sponge roller. Did the rest of my class perform this morning ritual? Before I even arrived at school, my hair had performed nothing short of a contortionist act. Bending, flipping, braided within its very self—all of this done, I imagine, to tame its rebellion and keep it from leaping and standing straight up on my head.

Little white fingers would touch my hair. During elementary school and before my family's move south, I was the only Black kid in my class, as there weren't many Black folks in Bristol, Connecticut. There were only two Black kids, myself and a mysterious fifth grader within my elementary school that I had never met. I remember seeing her while in line for lunch. She was a unicorn. I had heard tales of her existence, but I had never seen her in real life until that point. I didn't know her name. We smiled. She, too, had dark brown skin that existed within a sea of white faces. I'd examine her face. Her hair. Did she have roller marks also? Did her mama use the same pink potion that my mama used on my hair before school? Eventually, she would depart from the lunch line, grabbing a seat with her PB&J and fellow fifth graders. I would return to the cave of others.

My Blackness didn't feel like some extraordinary thing, of which I needed to be made aware. The only people who seemed to need an announcement were the non-Black people around me. I remember college being filled with White people who were surprised by my cosmos within their space. At times, occupying space felt liberating. I was no longer at home and could be who I wanted to be, wear whatever I wanted to wear, eat whatever I wanted to eat. I was grown, dammit, and my 250-square-foot dorm room was the Milky Way. However, the cosmos would reveal itself to be full of assumptions. I would feel the blow of supposition every time someone would create these assumptions around my upbringing. I remember their looks as they found out that I didn't come from a rough neighborhood. Although I had journeyed far from home, I was still in the South. The vast majority of White people who attended this school came from small towns, the Midwest, and places where very few folks looked like me. I think they had hoped that I had come from a neighborhood ravaged by gang violence. It would've been interesting. Different even. I would have been their teacher, educating them in the ways of the world from which I came.

I'll never forget visiting one of my college roommates' homes as we turned in to her suburban neighborhood. She glanced over at me in a way that was not so obvious but unmistakable. I knew what she was hoping. She was looking, searching for my reaction to their nicely manicured lawns and neatly placed mailboxes with tiny American flags. Finally, she looked over at me and asked the question that her face had already revealed. "Does your neighborhood look like this?" There was no shame to be found within her question or her face. This person was a friend of a friend that had now become my roommate. I could feel her studying the movement of my body. I guess she was searching for my eyes to light up at the sight of her suburban treasure. She wanted me to ooh and aah over her gated community, symmetric front yard landscaping, and dark oak doors that seemed to match my skin perfectly. Did she ooh and aah over it too? At that moment, I realized that I was her Black friend. At that moment, I felt no different than the brown oak doors that stood front and center within her neighborhood. They, too, were there for all to see.

She repeated the question as if I hadn't heard her, "So does your neighborhood look like this?" My head said, "Stop." My mouth said, "Yep." This girl had no clue that I was very familiar with this neighborhood. That my parents presently resided in this neighborhood.

Growing up, I tasted a variety of boroughs. I was born in Connecticut and grew up in Alabama. I lived in a majority-Black neighborhood, and then by high school lived in a majority-White area. By the time I was in college, I had lived everywhere and nowhere in between. This world and country were my community. I belonged everywhere and nowhere. For anyone who has felt unseen, the dismissal, the casting out, an oceanic feeling of being othered, it is with this spirit that I write this chapter.

The othering feels like tiny cuts above the skin's surface that no one can see or touch. There is no raised bruising or keloid marks, only callousness and hardness that has been exacted and weighed upon the shoulders of its lucky recipient. The othering robs us of our humanity, stifling the dealer's ability to show empathy for one's experience. The othering is transmitted not only across our skin, gender, and sexuality, but also our feelings, our emotions, and the quiet rage that has to stay like so. Quiet. Like many who have felt the pain of othering's sting, it doesn't begin with one moment, nor does it end after the moment subsides. It often happens throughout our lives. In this skin, our sex, toward our bodies, wafting all around, attempting to put us all "in our place."

My experience with othering began long before Trump, before insurrections and the return of abortion bans. As a child, I felt the othering by the stares I received in the South, the assumptions about my background due to the color of my skin, and so much more. As an adult, the hope was that this country could, should be better. It seemed that up until the 2016 election, our cries had gone unheard. For us, 2016 brought no shock. America was birthed and reared in trauma and had yet to heal from it. Perhaps all of America would now be in on what so many of us knew to be true. The truth being that Black lives don't seem to matter until White lives do.

After the election, I remember dropping Jax off at school and seeing White women hugging, even crying. I felt empathy. I did. I imagine that if I possessed the privilege to have somehow missed what had been going on since America's conception and was just now tuning in to this shit show of a horror movie, perhaps I, too, would have been terrified. Maybe. Seeing these women openly grieving saddened me. I hadn't witnessed this level of grief over the atrocities that had occurred during the killings of numerous unarmed men and women of color by law enforcement. It would have been nice to see these same women hugging and consoling one another following the murders of Sandra Bland or Korryn Gaines. Were Sandra and Korryn not their sisters?

Even now, as we hear of Trump running again for president, I am in voluntary denial. In the back of my mind, I know it has happened and could happen again. I know that history might repeat itself, walking backward into the gloaming, for lack of a better word. But I just can't believe it. And still I root for America and her ability to gift the equitable opportunity to provide a life of true freedom for everyone here. However, I know in my heart of hearts that she, too, may be like an emotionally ill-equipped parent who won't, can't, give what they don't or perhaps never had, and Trump is merely her son to whom was passed down the blueprint of this country's heritage.

I often imagine running away with my family to a distant land, another country, where there are fewer cases of hostility, bigotry, and phobias rooted in hate. I imagine a world without fear and racially induced weathering as I raise my children and cultivate my sacred happiness and theirs. We, too, know the secret that our ancestors knew long ago. They knew we must run to our joy, safe spaces, and ultimately our freedom. We must run to the places where we are seen in our beautiful humanity. Please know that it is not that I don't believe Trump and those like him can't be elected now or in the future, and that somehow America has learned her lesson. But part of my thriving while othered is imagining how I can make our world more unrestrained regardless of those who wish they could bottle up our bodies, sexual orientation, skin, and other characteristics. My thriving is actively moving toward the beauty surrounding us while also knowing the ugly bias that lives here. I am rooting for America to do better, *and* I am rooting for those of us who have felt the sting of being othered and our rightful place in the seat of thriving.

Resist, they said.
Stay woke, they said.
Have you read the paper today? It's all over the news.
It's everywhere. Little did they know.
I had been resisting since birth.
My very ethos and existence was an act of resistance. My joy,
  as well.

We saw the othering played out right in front of our eyes with the killing of George Floyd; as ex–police officer and now convict Derek Chauvin knelt on George's neck as he cried out for his mother. His pleas and cries meant nothing to this officer. He failed to see that George was somebody's father, kinfolk, friend or lover, somebody's baby, and most important, a stakeholder in the human race. I remember feeling the othering while watching clips of the trial on my screen. I couldn't bring myself to watch it in its entirety. Hope and fear were instant. The othering produced awareness that those who wrote the laws knew that they were not formed with me or those who looked like me in mind. These rules that were meant to protect and serve were not meant to preserve nor help me. And it is because of this knowledge that I would experience moments of uncertainty and the holding of my breath as if it were bittersweet fruit. I held my breath close like a newborn babe, fragile and in need of care. Sure, the evidence was clear that murder had taken place in the death of George Floyd. However, we had seen how this plays out in a not-so-distant past and very present history. Because of this, my breath felt like a prized possession. I would let it go and exhale when I thought it safe to do so, and only then.

The rules and safety apply to some, and not to those of us who are considered "other." We witnessed as insurrectionists stormed the United States Capitol on January 6, 2021. We watched as people scaled the building, broke into its chambers, and threatened to "take back" their country. Many marginalized groups marveled yet were unsurprised by their boldness as this act of treason unfolded. There was no shock at the privilege of Whiteness taking place. We knew the spoken and evident truth that marginalized groups would have been killed on sight by the Capitol Police. These boundaries of safekeeping were not threaded together in our heads by pure imagination. They were built within the fabric of the country.

The Palm

When I think of how we have been made to feel othered, I am reminded of the palm. I purchased my first palm a few years ago. It was around my mother's birthday, and I wanted to invite some lavish greenery into our home. This palm would be the first of the many plants that I would adopt. I named my new palm Agnes. For a while, Agnes seemed to be doing well. I mean, she wasn't dead. So there was that. I was new to plant life. Back then, my success would be measured by whether my plant was simply alive and not approaching death's door. Truth be told, while my beloved Agnes wasn't dying, she also wasn't growing.

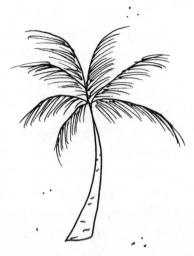

Eventually, I would come across the culprit. Mealybugs. Mealybugs are precisely as annoying as they sound. They are tiny, fuzzy insects that bear a resemblance to cotton balls. Mealybugs feed off the nutrients in plant juices, leaving behind a sticky powdery secretion. This pest drains and then craps on whatever plant it chooses to possess.

The mealybugs had ravaged Agnes. These fuzzy little fuckers had begun to eat and ultimately destroy my dear sweet palm. They would attack and deplete her, stripping her of any nutrients at the point of contact where maturation would occur. I was under the broad assumption that Agnes would take care of herself, which is a valid reason I chose her. She was strong and self-sufficient. All I had to do, I thought, was sit her by a window and give her a drink of water now and then. I realized at this moment that in my negligence of failing to check in on her, these tiny little invaders had not only depleted her but cut short her innate ability to do what plants do . . . grow. Because of these mealybugs (and my lack of care), Agnes was not growing into the whole and lush indoor palm she could be.

My options? I could go leaf by leaf, starting from the root up, and wipe away the pests using neem oil or rubbing alcohol, or I could begin pruning. I could cut her leaves back past the bugs and her sun-scorched brown spots and start over so that Agnes could realize her ontogeny. I opted to prune her back. I needed to protect her growth.

POC have had to flourish in spaces not designed for us or with us in mind, like my palm. Spaces that were even created for our destruction and overall failure, requiring that we shield ourselves from anything that acts as a disruption to our joy, peace, and general best state of health and ability to be well. But, much like the palm, we thrive anyway.

Cultivating Joy While Othered

Dear reader, when thriving while being othered, be it by race, disability, size, gender, or sexuality, we must pay attention to our body's signals and triggers. Asking ourselves where it hurts and touching that space to heal. Centering self-care, mental health, joy, and emotional well-being is essential. When people say Black Lives Matter, it means our entire lives matter—our joy, peace, creativity, and health. All of it matters. You matter even when your name is not a hashtag.

So what does the centering look like? It begins with asking yourself, "What is it that I need to navigate, in my healthiest form, my family, this country, and this world?" It looks like a prioritization of therapy and working through trauma. For the record, when we talk about Black folks' reparations, I believe that free therapy should be part of the package, since the trauma that we have encountered, be it personally or even on a cellular level, requires all the support necessary for our thriving. Here lies the bridge to joy. This bridge is filled with intentional work.

You have felt expectation's weight of being strong, holding the world together, and lacking the privilege of falling apart. Dear reader, I ask that you take space, take time, and relish in peace. Do what births your highest joy. Choose yourself and your heart. The world, your family, your circles can wait.

> *Grow, girl, grow.*
> *Look at that soil, dark and rich.*
> *Earthworms and ladybugs are working*
>   *overtime. Sun is giving you warmth.*
> *Rain kissing your budding leaves.*
> *Lemons, tomatoes,*
> *Oak and ferns*
> *You are growing, girl . . . Just like them.*

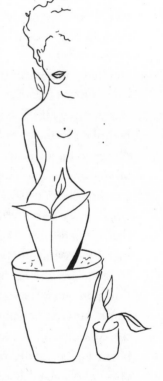

What is the mealybug? The mealybug is anything that attacks growth and induces depletion, anything that can rob you of your fullness. Your mealybug could be that social media account that leaves you feeling empty. What are you seeing and taking in through your eyes? For example, seeing POC gunned down by law enforcement on your timeline triggers anxiety on a cellular level. Taking in constant images of violence often engages cellular memory passed down, leaving us feeling overwhelmed, troubled, and afraid. Cellular or ancestral memory can only be described as that uncomfortable truth we feel in our bones, but we can't exactly put our finger on why. Some call it epigenetics. New studies have shown that experiences or trauma can be passed down cellularly, impacting subsequent generations.

When I became pregnant with our son Jupiter, I did a complete social media overhaul. I cleaned house. I deleted several Instagram accounts from my feed. Truthfully, I found myself in full alignment with a lot of these deleted accounts. However, being pregnant while Black and having the threat of being three to four times more likely to die during childbirth, being triggered was not something that I needed to add to the list. In this case, I opted to prune and cultivate my online usage. I also practiced this intentional pruning with entertainment, movies, and news articles.

When I was thirty-three weeks pregnant with Jupiter, I almost went into preterm labor. Jon was traveling quite a bit for work. I was wearing all the hats and firing on all cylinders. I began our bedtime routine of putting the boys to sleep in the evening and retreated to our living room, plopping my round pregnant body on the sofa. While there, I did what most folks do while on the couch. I decided to watch a movie. The movie of choice? *Roots.* I had never seen the film. Perhaps I felt that those who knew that fact would revoke my Black card. What if folks found out that I lacked a point of reference for the character "Chicken George," besides his being portrayed by Ben Vereen? I felt that this moment was as good as any. I sat there. I watched "Kunta Kinte" survive kidnapping, shackles, and a long boat ride across the Atlantic. While watching, I began to think of all the Black boys who looked like my Black boys being stolen from their parents, who looked like me. Where did they go? Their parents would never see their sons again. They would never see their daughters again. What about the parents who were stolen? The mothers? What about the child that was left behind, desperately searching for her mother's breast, a home that would never return?

I continued watching. I arrived at the scene in the film where an enslaved woman dies during childbirth. She dies in the cotton fields, with her oppressor standing over her, whip in hand. Instantly, and almost as if our bodies were in sync, I begin to have painful contractions. I was afraid and only thirty-three weeks along. Jon was traveling. I wanted to have a home birth. If I went into labor now, birthing at home would be out of the question. I thought to myself, this can't happen now. I called Jon. Jon called my midwife, Racha. My midwife called me. She asked, "What were you doing?" I responded, "Nothing." Within the hour, my dear friend Andrea came over. She put the kids to bed. She also put me to bed. I went to sleep with the contractions now dulled with time and my worry of an impending labor decreased.

The next day, my midwife and I touched base. I realized at that moment that I hadn't been candid with her when she inquired regarding what I had been doing before the previous night's scare. It was a truth that didn't come easy. I was taking on and taking in too much. Feelings of overwhelm and shame caused me to give pause about coming clean. I knew better. I'm a birth worker. Taking space and reclaiming one's time is the ethos by which I live. If I were to share my truth, my midwife would discover my hypocrisy. Sure, I wasn't moving furniture, rearranging my home, or doing some strenuous task that could seem like the cause for possible preterm labor contractions. However, what was I watching? I had no other choice but to admit it. I told her I was watching *Roots*. She didn't judge me. However, she did ask why. My reply: "I'd never watched it before. I figured, why not?" Without a pause, she responded with two words—cellular memory. She explained that while I have never personally experienced the bitter taste of slavery, more than likely my great-great-great-grandmother had. Perhaps I shared memories similar to the enslaved woman dying in the blood- and sweat-stained cotton fields. Maybe my great-great-

great-grandmother had seen women die in the same Alabama heat. Toil, blood, fear, and pain intermingle as they birth their babies into an evil, cruel, dark Southern world. History passed down these memories on a cellular level. Perhaps, just perhaps, I remembered a scene similar to this in a place that can't be seen, but instead remembered in the deep and untouched. Only felt. From then on (or at least for the duration of my pregnancy), my show of choice would be *Modern Family*.

ANCESTRAL MEMORY

A dear colleague of mine, Dr. Cleopatra Kamperveen, refers to this ancestral memory and affirms our power to alter the degree of expression of our genetics being passed down through epigenetics. This idea bucks against the thought that our genetic inheritance is our final destiny. She references epigenetics' root word when describing its possibilities—"epigenetics" means "above genetics." Dr. Kamperveen shares within her fertility practice the concept of the Primemester period, a magical time wherein birthing people have the ability and power to dial into their genetic strengths and dial back their genetic vulnerabilities. The Primemester is the first 120-plus days before conception. Dr. Kamperveen mentions that we must create safety during this time, address underlying trauma, and strip away everything that leaves us emotionally depleted before conception. By tapping into epigenetics, you can change the genetic inheritance of your children, grandchildren, and in some cases, up to seven generations.

You do not have to birth a child to participate in this ancestral prep work. When othered, we can be our very own soft and safe places when in the Primemester of our goal conception. Here's how:

1. **Address our underlying trauma,** becoming curious about how it affects our ability to actualize our pursuits. Do you often believe there's no room at the table for you? Do you feel like an impostor in spaces where you are more than qualified? I think this is where othering and trauma often meet. Remember, othering and not belonging can go hand in hand. Until we disrupt it, that is. **Affirm with me: I can feel othered *and* still belong *right here*.**

2. **Strip away everything that leaves us emotionally depleted** before conception. Although initially subtle, the mealybug is there to suck out every bit of nutrient for survival.

A mealybug can be that person who lacks awareness of your current capacity. I remember running to the grocery store with the boys. As we were getting out of the car, a woman approached us and began telling us about how much she just loved "us"— how she just loved our skin, and so on. She then went into this monologue on "oppression" and how Black men must fight the oppressor. It was overwhelming. After a couple of minutes of educating me on my people's state, she bade me farewell. I was left overloaded and exhausted. Here I was just trying to be a carefree Black woman shopping for kale, and suddenly I was bombarded by this overzealous character and her need to educate. At that moment, I realized that I would have to be intentional about protecting my joy not only against the dreaded racist but also against the newly "woke" people who had little to no concern for the capacity with which I could hold their unloading. This lady didn't care about me or my being. She just wanted to prove to me all that she had learned. She didn't care that up until that point, my sons and I had been having a relaxing day, shopping for groceries, as regular people do. She didn't care about my sons. She didn't care that they were enjoying their childhood, safely under the protective wing of their mama bird. Thanks to Whole Foods Wendy, I now had to have a different conversation with my eldest that included oppression and other-ing objectification instead of the lighter dialogue of "What's for dinner tonight?"

A mealybug can be that person or thought that deprives you of the right to be human and simply exist. I call it "goddess syndrome."

As a Black woman, I have been called a "goddess" more times than I would like to or can imagine. Truthfully, I see many a flaw with this term. It robs us Black women of our humanity and plays into the strong Black woman archetype, an ethos that has run Black women into the ground since forever. The goddess syndrome is a crime that's been committed far too often. When we are not seen as a threat or the "angry Black woman," we are seen as magical. Mythical. The oracle even. Or worse, "goddess." This monolithic otherworldly attribution can cause depletion. **Affirm with me: I have the right to be simply human, accompanied by all the beauty that it entails.**

Sure, I am all about #BlackGirlMagic. However, there are days in which I feel more Black Girl than Magic. Like other humans, I, too, get overwhelmed and exhausted. There are days when I need space and room to grow, safe spaces where I am not consumed and spit out. You too?

There are days when I, too, need to yell and not bite my tongue due to fear of being labeled as aggressive or, worse, angry. Yet, as a goddess, I am deprived of this human gift.

I'll never forget Hannah. Hannah was a postnatal client of mine. Hannah had just given birth to a new baby girl. I was one of her many postpartum doulas. She had the means to afford around-the-clock support. I recall meeting her for the first time. She had her babe at her breast. Both were cozy and snuggled in bed. She seemed kind. She was articulate and educated. One could tell that she prided herself on her many accomplishments. She spoke calmly and sweetly as her little one nestled close. She called me a goddess.

I had just brought up a freshly cooked meal for her to devour. My love language is cooking. I had prepared eggs cooked in ghee. Avocado. Fresh fruit. She breathlessly replied, "Thank you," and then she referred to me as a goddess again. Although those words hit me in a place that felt off, I thought nothing of it. I released it. After all, it was a compliment. A few days later, I was not only doing the regular day-to-day tasks that most birth workers do; I found myself driving Hannah around. I felt like Morgan Freeman in the film *Driving Miss Daisy*. I began staying long past the hours within our original agreement. I was getting yelled at and then apologized to by Hannah.

I remember holding her little one as she pumped. Her baby was crying as my milk began to leak. At the time, I was knee-deep in breastfeeding my middle son, Jedi. Hannah looked at me and became visibly upset. I asked her what was wrong, desperately wanting to hold space. She said that she felt terrible. I assumed that she would say that she felt awful that I was here with her and her babe while my babe was home. Instead, she said she referred to my milk-making capabilities and her struggle therewith. At that moment, I remembered the word "goddess," a term that she had thrown my way numerous times. A name that had not quite landed comfortably. Now I knew why. She didn't see me as human. She didn't see me as anything outside of her world. She was upset because I, whom she'd viewed as a "goddess," could seemingly do it all. Truthfully, one could argue that most new parents cannot see beyond their current postpartum world. Trust me, I've been there. Also, as a doula, it is our job to leave the outside world on the outside. However, I've seen and experienced people like Hannah. They are the same people who only see bodies with skin like mine as an asset. Nothing more. The same person will ask Oprah or Michelle Obama to run for president as if they are nothing unless they are everything to everyone. I am not a goddess, nor is any person who seems to have strong shoulders and an ancestral history of bearing the weight on their back. We are humans with human emotions and needs.

IDENTIFY YOUR MEALYBUG

How do we thrive within this shell, our body, this skin?

We first identify the mealybug. As mentioned, your mealybug can be anything that depletes you, deprives you of your humanity and the tenderness you deserve. The palm tree can grow lush and full. However, its growth can be cut short by tiny little pests. We must take a pause and check in with ourselves so that the mealybug will lack the opportunity to choke out our happiness, peace, and, most notably, our realization of our best selves.

This checking-in looks like asking ourselves these three questions:

1. Is it oppressive, or does it support my liberation?
2. Does it create disorder or aid in my whole body well-being?
3. Is it mine to carry, or is it mine to release?

By checking in, I can dismantle the "strong Black woman" ethos and grant myself an allowance to lean into softness, vulnerability, and community. Becoming aware of the pests that rob us of our vitality is essential, as when we see them and recognize them as such, we can then allow those things to go in grace, calling forth the right to bloom, blossom, and harvest everything that we need to thrive.

IDENTIFY YOUR RESISTANCE

What is your unique gifting to your community and yourself? I believe it's important to know what you can offer within the space you occupy. Otherwise, we may try to be all the things to everyone, which is impossible. We must be ever conscious that changing the space in which we occupy as a whole is the result of a larger problem. A problem that will not get solved in a day or with positive thoughts, well wishes, or even this book. The broader issue is systemic racism in such areas as conventional educational systems and standardized testing, historical redlining, food deserts, environmental racism, the school-to-prison pipeline, and institutional design. This problem began generations ago and is written into our Constitution's very language.

During the racial uprising of 2020, many folks found their way and their act of resistance within this historical moment. Some marched, protested, rioted. Many voted and wrote letters to their elected officials, letting their voices be heard. I wanted to march. However, we were knee-deep in a global pandemic during this time, and I had three kids at home. I needed to keep myself safe and well, not only for my children but also for the newborn babies that I would welcome into the world as a birth guide. So, in that season of necessary racial upheaval, my resistance was being present with my three Black boys and making sure that they knew that they were safe within our home. National Guard tanks would drive past our house. I would close the curtains, put on music, and diffuse lavender, assuring my boys that we were okay, although the outside world was a literal dumpster fire. As sirens blared on by and their nervous system felt activated in ways they had never been before, I reminded them to find home within their bodies and our arms. I reminded them that they were protected and sound and that their mama and papa—well, "We got you." We let them stay up past their bedtime as curfews were put into place all over the city and cop cars and ambulances whizzed by. We watched movies and snuggled them close. Outside was chaos. Inside was joy. Mothering my three Black boys and keeping their minds and my body healthy and safe was my resistance.

Find Your North

We thrive by finding our north. A dear sister-friend of mine and author, Kimberly Seals-Allers, spoke of sending her children to London to live with their father during the pandemic, and more specifically, during the continued racial pandemic and uprising of 2020. She shared that when weighing her options for her children's safety, she was confident that her son would more than likely survive if he contracted Covid. However, she questioned his chances of surviving the escalated racism within our country. Kimberly experienced anxiety like most Black mothers raising young Black children. Her instinct was to stay put and fight on another day in hopes of this world getting better, being better. However, she remembered our ancestors who risked life and limb to head north to find safety and solace, to find freedom. And just like those who came before us, we too have the right to find our north. To find and occupy spaces of safety, wholeness, and freedom. Reminiscent to your life, your emotional safety matters, and when this reality feels questionable or nonprioritized, you have the right to advocate and run toward that safety.

We who have been made to feel shame around our bodies
Full body and slim
Gay, Queer, Trans
Disabled
Woman
POC
Wherever you find yourself within the spectrum of castaway.
I want you to know that you have the right to feel safe.

During the aftermath of the George Floyd protests worldwide, black squares filled our social media timelines. We saw beautiful online moments of the dominant culture sharing the mic and their respective platforms. However, I'll never forget this one company that approached me and asked that I share my experience within the motherhood community as a Black mother and expert within my field. At first, this sounded interesting, until my internal teacher presented pause, and I shortly after knew why. While the organization explained their objective, they mentioned that they would provide an opportunity and "safe space" for their community to ask me any question they would like without fear of judgment, even racist questions. The company's objective was to create "a safe space" for their majority White community to be curious about my Black experience within this world. However, where was the "safe space" for me? Within that moment, I chose to use this as an opportunity to let them know how this request of me to answer uncensored questions was not only problematic but emotionally violent. I told them that they had a severe blind spot exposed, as my safety didn't even register as a priority, while instead, their White community's curiosity took precedence over the possibility of my Black discomfort or even danger.

Attempting to explain your humanity can, and will, never take the place of the nonmarginalized taking personal accountability, inventory, and gathering themselves instead of expecting the marginalized to do it for them. You reserve the right to refuse to offer any part of yourself that jeopardizes your physical and emotional safety, that doesn't support your joy, autonomy, and purpose. Dearest reader, you have the right to say no to anything that doesn't feel right, doesn't align, or doesn't contribute to your thriving. You don't even have to know why. You can go on a mere hunch. You have the right to listen to your body and what's coming from the teacher within, channel Sophia from *The Color Purple,* and give a strong "Hell no!" Locate the safe (and the unsafe) areas within your world, so that when the weight of being other feels too cumbersome to bear, you too can head north to a place of protection. Identify the moments, people, and most important, the internal factors that allow you to feel seen and grounded.

We thrive by knowing ourselves. Know when to prune and pull back. We mentioned pruning in the previous chapters in regard to relationships. The same is true with self. Like my palm, we must know when it is needed to pull back, to prune so that we can bloom into our whole selves. If you fall within the marginalized category, you are conditioned to work harder. It is essential to know when things feel too much, and when they do, cut away those elements holding us down and getting in the way.

Last, find your light. Find the places that nourish you and run to them. Locate the warm, inviting spaces where you are honored and seen. Where your magic and ordinary are held within the same love and appreciation. This light may come from community groups and like-minded friends whose company breathes life into your cells. Please, I implore you to find this healing glow. And when you can't find said light, perhaps you are the one to create it.

One of the many things that I love about plants is their will and determination to live by any means necessary. Have you ever noticed your plant unapologetically reaching for the sun? One of my favorite plants is my philodendron selloum plant, Dinah. I've had her comfortably seated near my east-facing window, as her leaves preside over a Kimberly fern, a prayer plant, and a cactus. Her long winding roots spill out of her pot and onto the floor. I often glance over at her and admire her bravery. What if we all dared not only to reach for the sun but to take up space while doing so?

I know. For most marginalized groups, we've been told that it's not okay. We've been told to shrink. Be less than our whole selves. How dare we reach over and beyond to kiss sunlight simply? How dare we be so bold? One of the many lessons I have learned from Dinah is that we must be brave anyway. Kiss the sun anyway, because our health and longevity depend on it. This fearless intimacy means stretching high and arriving in the exact place where we've always belonged—deeply rooted in self-worth. When we are aware of our worth, the question shifts from how dare we be so bold to why would we not? Why would we not ask for that promotion? Why would we not take that vacation? Why would we not take up all the space within our universe? When in doubt, be like Dinah.

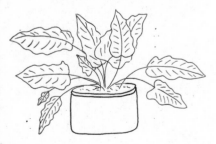

1. **How are you creating ritual?** When othered, how do you remain tethered to community and care?

2. **Identify your resistance.** For *you,* what does resistance look like?

3. **Are mealybugs present?** Once they are identified, how can you begin pruning?

4. **Find your north.** Where can you find solace while othered?

CHAPTER THIRTEEN

Rest—It's for You

The day was long.

After completing her shift, I imagine she packed her bags from her work locker, changed out of her uniform, gathered her keys, and walked to her car. Perhaps her partner picked her up from work, or maybe she had driven herself that day. I often wonder if they had made plans earlier that morning for what they would do for dinner. Perhaps there were plans for the weekend. I imagine her gathering her things, waving goodbye to her colleagues as she headed home. One of them would possibly say something funny as she rolled down the window of her car. She would ask them to repeat it. After which, they would both share a laugh. After all, the day was long, and laughter was what she needed to end her day. I see her taking a deep sigh as she waves goodbye to her colleagues, promising to see them tomorrow.

She had spent her day in and out of her office on wheels, as an EMS worker receiving calls over the communication system, speeding to locations and people who required help. Receiving calls that ranged from something as simple as acute distress to more life-or-death situations couldn't have been easy. I would think that it might raise one's stress levels in unimaginable ways. However, this was her job, and like many who had the honor to serve surrounding communities, I would guess that it was more than likely something of which she was proud. I envision her riding home, reflecting on her day. Remembering the people she had helped, kept from dying, and the ones that didn't make it, and her heart ripping into a million pieces as she pondered how she could have helped more, although she had given it her all. I think of her wanting to do a "good job." Whatever that meant. She wanted to do her best. I envision her thinking of her mother and the times she reminded her to do the best that she could because the world would more than likely judge her most harshly. The world was cold. However, I like to think of her reflecting on her mama's words, and those words feeling like a warm washing of grace and truth.

I think of her as a little Black girl seated between her mother's legs as she, too, parted her hair straight down the middle and then into pigtails. I see her mother greasing her scalp and anointing her head with oil for the road ahead. I dream of her mother holding her chocolate face between her hands, holding her face close as she would kiss her goodbye on the way to school, summer camp, or simply goodnight.

Perhaps she and her partner had plans when she got home. I want to think that they did. Maybe they ordered in. After all, she had been out all day being a modern-day superhero. When deciding what to order, I would think that they went through the motions of the winning choice. Like many couples going back and forth only to settle on the same meal they always eat, I think of them. Perhaps when the food arrived, they sat on the sofa eating and laughing at their favorite TV show. Or maybe they took it outside, sat on the front of the car, and counted the stars. I think that whatever they chose, they were happy. I hope that they were happy. I think of her sharing complex parts of her day and the parts that filled her cup to the brim. I imagine her partner listening and being happy for her too.

After eating, they would wash dishes together. Or perhaps they would skip the dishes altogether. After all, it had been a long day. She was tired. She would put on her pajamas, maybe an old T-shirt she had slept in since high school. I imagine her and her partner staring at each other in bed and laughing and perhaps joking about how exhausted they both were. Her partner would share about his day, how maybe the people on his job were a pain in the ass. They would laugh and eventually drift off to sleep.

This moment would be the last time Breonna Taylor would go to sleep or wake up, the last time that she would laugh, share a joke with a friend, pack her bags after a long day at work. Share a tender moment with her partner. This moment would be the last time she lay down to rest.

I'll never forget hearing about Breonna Taylor, a twenty-six-year-old Black woman murdered in her home by police as she slept. It was now apparent that resting or sleeping was another thing Black people could not do without the fear of death. Breonna was sleeping in her bed when she was gunned down, just as Botham Jean, a twenty-six-year-old Black Dallas accountant who was leisurely smoking a joint and eating ice cream on his sofa, resting, when an officer barged in and fatally shot him—resting while Black activated me for weeks. Before going to bed, I would make sure that I locked all of the doors and that all the curtains were closed, as if somehow this checklist would keep me and mine safe while sleeping. The message was clear: Black folks couldn't even rest without fear of what might happen to them, and what would never happen to those with lighter skin.

I wasn't the only one activated in this way. Many Black Americans felt the threat somatically. The idea that someone could barge in, guns drawn, was not only maddening but terrifying. Within this time, I began to lean into the idea of *rest as resistance,* feeling that perhaps it could also be a method for thriving. With the spirit of resistance and those who are now ancestors, I write this chapter for Breonna, Botham, and those who worked the fields from sunup to sundown, only to sleep and not experience rest.

It is hard to think about Breonna Taylor and Botham Jean and not go further back. Back to a time my ancestors also held many of the same fears as Black Americans today. While writing this book, I telephoned my grandmother, Juril. I was curious to see rest through her eyes and whether, and how, it had meshed or perhaps revised through time. My grandmother shared how she and her family lived on Sunrise Hill in Sylacauga, Alabama. Her mother, my great-grandmother Mama Dear, grew up with her brothers and sisters in the mid-1920s working the fields and cleaning houses to make ends meet and put food on the table. My great-grandmother and her siblings had lost their parents early. Mama Dear lost her father suddenly to a stroke and her mother to what they believe to be diabetes, as she'd ask for a slice of "cooked bread" just so that she could make it home from the fields each day and not collapse on the walk. After the death of their parents, the siblings were raised by their stepfather. After the older siblings were old enough to care for the younger siblings, they all set out on their own, escaping the abuse of their stepfather and finding love and protection amongst each other.

Mama Dear and her siblings worked the land. They were employed by two kind White men, Mr. Watson and Mr. Stone. These men paid the young people a living wage and assisted them in acquiring and purchasing land, which my family still owns to this day. One day, a police officer barged into the home of Mama Dear's brother, my great-uncle Buddy. They broke in unannounced while he was in bed recovering from measles. The officers grabbed Uncle Buddy out of bed after receiving reports that a Black man had committed an offense. Because the siblings had all built homes on their newly purchased land within a stone's throw of one another, my great-grandmother and her siblings heard and saw the commotion. The police continued to pull my uncle out of his bed as he pleaded, feverishly confused by what was taking place. The police officer barging into my great-uncle's home, with or without cause, could have resulted in near-death beatings or lynching. Either way, Mama Dear wasn't having it. The story goes that after witnessing what the officer was attempting to do, she began swinging her arms and beating the cop's ass. By the time it was said and done, she had not only beat him black and blue, but she had also stripped him down to his boxers and taken his pistol. As the police officer called for backup, and the siblings heard the sound of more police cars in the distance, my great-aunt Louise begged and pleaded for Mama Dear to get in the car to get away because God knows what could happen to a Black woman who had done what she had.

Mama Dear and Uncle Buddy were arrested and taken to the small-town jail. As she waited in the cell, the police officer whom she'd beaten silly tried to come in. And in true fashion, she reminded him of what had already been done to him and what she was capable of doing if he entered the cell and tried to harm her family again. She looked him square in the eyes. Her words were, "Come in here if you want to. I'll stick your head in that commode." She had already proved to him that she wasn't afraid. He believed her.

Meanwhile, her siblings back home rushed and told Mr. Watson and Mr. Stone what had just transpired. The men phoned down to the station, calling for the immediate release of Mama Dear and Uncle Buddy or else. They told the precinct over the phone, "If the Morrises are not released immediately and outside the precinct on the sidewalk by the time we arrive to pick them up, there will be hell to pay." These two men, Mr. Watson and Mr. Stone, had influence and the currency of Whiteness, which they used for good. My great-grandmother and great-uncle were outside waiting for Mr. Watson and Mr. Stone to pick them up when they arrived, safe, sound, and undefeated.

They would work from sunup to sundown, cultivating collard greens and harvesting yams, bell peppers, and all the fruits and vegetables they could muster. Rest was a thing that they only obtained after they completed a day's work. For Black folks back then, Sunday was their day of rest. My grandmother and her siblings would walk down the hill to Shiloh Baptist Church, where their family and those before them retreated to worship and form community. Knees and ankles were well-greased. The oiling of ashy knees felt reminiscent of the anointing of Jesus as Mary Magdalene used her last bit of oil, the women of my family and Mary both using what they had on their beloved. Black folks found rest in the laying on of hands by mothers as they prepared their children for church. Rest was found in the greasing of ankles and hair separation like the Red Sea before Sunday School. Hair slicked, tamed, and oiled. Each child taking turns, as they would get their face lotioned, as Mama Dear would not so delicately rub cocoa butter on their cocoa-colored cheeks, with the determination that only Black mothers possess. Frilled socks, church shoes, dresses, and Sunday suits in child form walked hand in hand as they made their Sunday march to the church house behind their mother.

In the summer of 1945, my great-grandmother lost her partner, my great-grandfather Frank Williams. Although she was only four years old when she lost her father, my grandmother remembers him. I listened to my grandmother as she described her father. How handsome he was, how he always wore white button-down shirts, and how his acquired nickname was Snow. And although no one knew how he earned this nickname, I like to think it was because he was just that cool. My great grandfather, Frank Williams, had dark skin, the color of the brownest tree trunk, the shade of the darkest brown of autumn leaves.

Many of the men back then for recreation would spend Friday nights congregating and having a good time. Friday nights were for gathering together, shooting dice, and drinking White Lightning. I hear the sound of Black men laughing and interrogating each other's fables. I listen to them saying "Shiiiiiiiiiit" in utter disbelief or disapproval depending on the subject matter. Dice would roll and hit the wall as both cheers and groans moved across the room. My great-grandfather would loosen his tie and roll up his sleeves as he rolled. He'd tug at his pants leg as he knelt on one knee before rolling the dice. This gathering of men, hoping to release the pressure of living in a cold-blooded world that hated their skin, was their comfort and release.

Friday nights were reserved for broad and boisterous laughs as Sundays were for restful sacred practice. Both Friday nights and Sunday mornings were holy and sacred spaces that offered a sense of rest from my great-grandparents' exhausting and frightening environment. They found rest in talking shit on a Friday night, in sharing Sunday dinner, in family. Much like Sunday morning, they found rest in the communion of White Lightning on Friday nights, the sexual hymns of Ma Rainey, and nicknames without origin because the knowledge of that nickname meant something peaceful. It was a secret password to familiarity, comfort, and home within the individual. However, back then, rest was earned after and only after the work was complete. If our theology around rest had an origin story, this would be it. Passed down generationally like hand-me-downs. You must earn your rest. Work for it, and then you can taste it until . . .

Where did you inherit your beliefs around rest?

Rest is healing and therapeutic.
We all thrive best when we have it.
Rest is our birthright.
Take it.

INTENTIONAL REST

Both the inherited ideas about rest and the very present anxiety over safety in leisure can often impede on our ability to carve out intentional rest. Stories of Breonna Taylor, Botham Jean, and my great-uncle Buddy, all seeking the fundamental right to rest while being deprived of it, are all true stories, and all individually create a somatic mark in how safe we feel while doing so. We subscribe to the belief that we must work first and then enjoy rest in our bodies. And yet and still, even when the work is done, we don't fully feel deserving of its open-armed welcome. This exclusion from rest sits with us. Yes, it sits with you and me both.

We must examine our rest. There is a distinction between sleep and rest, and knowing the difference between the two is fundamental to our thriving. Rest is the greatest deactivation or the radical ability and demand to power our systems down. Unlike sleep, rest is not automatic. It is a skill to be seized and then embodied. When we think of rest in this way, we can carry it with us when we sleep and even in our waking state throughout. We all sleep; however, resting can feel unattainable and never entirely within our grasp. While living in these bodies can create the highest joy, the unkind world can produce the weariness that so many marginalized people experience. To walk into a room and be the only _____ there can put our nervous system in a state of activation. Whether in our workplace or our place of worship, we are activated, even if unconsciously. We feel the need to say the right things in these spaces. Fear is present, as is our cellular memory and awareness of survival. After a long day of living in a heightened sense of attention, the vigilance does not end. To be othered while waking or sleeping is to be in a constant state of somatic activation.

In the past, intentionally resting has been hard for me. For starters, I have never enjoyed napping. Don't get me wrong—once in bed, I have never had a hard time falling asleep or sleeping in general. However, *intentionally resting* has always been a hard sell. I remember as a young kid feeling as if I was somehow missing out on the fun happening on the other side of my bedroom's closed door. There were still adventures to be had, and I wanted in on them. Truthfully, this FOMO (fear of missing out) would continue well into adulthood as my fear of having not done enough to earn said rest also developed. Until recent years, I had filed this angst against napping into the "Well, that's just the way I am" folder. In reality, this fear of resting was deeply rooted in the need to prove and be approved. I like to call it the hustle syndrome. I'm sure many parents, Black folks, women, and most marginalized groups feel it.

As someone who checks all the above boxes (Black, Woman, Mother, and more), I felt this pressure triple the load. I worked harder because it was never enough. I'd feel the tightness and anxiety building as I raced to exceed deadlines and expectations because if I didn't, that meant failure. Learning to prioritize one's self-care above all else has required that I unlearn the toxic expectations of powering through. It has required that I understand that my body, my mental health, and my life as a whole matter. When we talk about liberation, we must include rest. Resting is where we cultivate our dreams, build our legacy, and sustain ourselves so that we can continue to thrive.

In the dirt, we grow.
In the dark, we grow.
Both are essential.

After the Civil War and during the Reconstruction era, lawmakers put Black Codes, racially discriminatory laws, in place. For the formerly enslaved it enacted laws that were purposefully used to limit the rights of freedmen and -women. Southern states had the right to enact and mandate laws limiting the formerly enslaved, stifling their freedoms. Although they were free, there was no liberty, let alone a pursuit of happiness.

Section 5 of the Mississippi Black Codes reads, "Every freedman, free negro and mulatto shall, on the second Monday of January, one thousand eight hundred and sixty-six, and annually thereafter, have a lawful home or employment, and shall have written evidence thereof . . ." In other words, Black folks had to provide proof of employment for the upcoming year, and if they did not, they could be charged with vagrancy, resulting in imprisonment. Parents were arrested and charged with vagrancy under these Southern codes and their children were allowed to be taken away and placed in "apprenticeships," which was just code for having another master. Children were placed within White homes, "places of employment," and forced to work as apprentices until the age of twenty-one for boys and eighteen for girls. Black Codes also prohibited gathering without permission from one's employer.

The Black Code continued throughout the Jim Crow era and into 1965. Post-slavery, we were forced to work. Allow that to sink in. From the time Black people arrived in this country, slave traders brought us here to work. And after we were technically freed, our work and rest were still regulated, forcing us to continue within the cycle. Knowing and sitting with this allows two things to be accurate and present:

- My work is not my worth.
- My work became my worth, not because of my own doing.

Knowing these two things will require intentional undoing.

REST AS LIBERATION

Our liberation is centered on our rest. I like to think of the seedling when imagining our flourishing. When we plant seeds in the ground, four things are necessary for the seed to grow. Our seed needs the proper environment consisting of temperature, air, light, and moisture. However, first we must determine the seed's needs according to the crop we are planting. A pepper seed's needs are different from an apple seed's needs. Once we have determined our seeds' specific blueprint, we can place them in the soil for growth.

One of the things that I find fascinating when planting is the need for balance. For example, our seed needs moisture. However, if we put too much water and compact the seed into the dirt, not enough air will get to the source, which will in turn prevent the seed from growing into the plant that we desire. There is also the balance of light and dark. Some seeds need more darkness than others. In fact, for some, resting in the dark is how they will mature from a tiny seed into a seedling, and exposing the seed to too much light too soon will prevent its maturation. These seeds know that resting in the environment needed is their ticket to becoming all they were created to be.

Regarding us humans, I like to think of our rest as our direct pathway to growth. Our environment, world, country, and ingrained culture play a specific part in our fruition. The toxic culture of staying busy and gathering our coins while sacrificing our mental and physical health is the antithesis of taking care and intentional rest. Our somatic response to navigating this world is to work harder. And I want you to know that it's not your fault. It is not your fault that you feel the need to prove your worth by your works. It's not your fault that simply doing nothing feels like idle hands, almost sinful. These are all things that have been inserted into our subconscious, cellular memory, and perception. However, I also want you to know that you are worthy of its unlearning.

My work became my worth and was placed within my cellular memory by breaking the backs of my ancestors. Like a candle, the light of worthiness was blown out as ink dried to paper, enforcing slavery, Black Codes, and Jim Crow laws. Unlearning that I must be constantly busy, creating, toiling, and giving until I am not only exhausted but depleted is the first key to thriving while being othered and the beginning of intentional rest. Exhaustion was one of the tools used to enslave and overwork as a wash and repeat, and to this day, depletion is still a tool used by our society to determine worthiness.

So how do we thrive while being othered? How do we move beyond the structures of our society that deem hustling the holy

grail? We take up rest as both our personal and collective resistance, unlearning and reframing our relationship with it. We
take a lesson from the seed.

As mentioned, the seed needs air, moisture, the right balance
of light and dark, and the perfect environment for that particular
seed to flourish into a seedling. If the seed does not receive
enough air, it simply cannot thrive. The same goes for us. We
often overextend ourselves, make sure that we are "keeping
busy," and ultimately do the most with the tiniest bit of rest in
the tank. We don't give ourselves enough air to breathe in our
environment. And anything that is living must have air.

I also think of how the seed must have the proper balance of
light and dark. We, too, must be okay with sitting and resting in
dark spaces. Most of the internal work we do, the unlearning, is
not done in the light but beneath the surface. Resting is a part of
the work, which I know can sound antithetical, but sometimes it
takes us looking at rest as a part of the process to thriving and
wholeness to even begin to prioritize it. Resting and sitting
within our fears as well as our inherited values are a part of our
germination. Many people have a hard time sitting within this
spot, as it is uncomfortable. Who wants to sit with the idea that
the beliefs around rest they've accumulated along the way no
longer serve them after so much toil? Who wants to sit with the
truth of why their ideas of working until they are parched bones
are perhaps only passed-down fears? I can only compare it to
discovering that there is no wizard behind the curtain but a
bone-tired, terrified human spreading these beliefs and fears to
all that will hear its message. We must do the work below the
surface so that when we grow and make our way aboveground,
we will not be scorched by the bright light of the sun—the bright
light of the sun being all the good that pours your way by way of
your talents and abilities. Without balance, producing more fruit

can feed the monster of needing more to satiate ourselves, which creates the nightmare of needing to toil more without rest. I want you to know that you can rest while sowing and harvesting. You can rest in all seasons.

Affirm with me: My worth is not found in my work or productivity. Working harder will never make me enough for others and especially myself.

Rest as Ritual

There are many benefits of a rest ritual. As mentioned, rest is not automatic for many, nor is it our natural reaction to our everyday environment. Rest is a skill and a purposeful practice holding many benefits.

When we center rest as a daily practice, we are less reactionary and more responsive. Your mood is balanced and less swayed by external stimuli. You may even find your thinking a bit clearer, and with less fear and anxiety.

What does a rest ritual look like practiced in everyday life?

It mirrors paying attention to where more ease and rest are needed. Where are the areas in your life where rest or deactivation is present? And then the opposite, be curious around when you feel most activated. Are you activated within your work and/ or familial environment? After watching news cycle after news cycle of triggering news? A rest ritual looks likes taking micro-moments throughout the day, reminding ourselves that we are safe. We can't always sit in the bathtub while sipping champagne or journey afar for our Eat, Pray, Love moment. I know. I wish we could too. Condensing our rest ritual on a practical and micro level can be precisely what the doctor ordered. Before entering the office, place one hand on your chest and the other on your belly, and breathe. Feel as all the parts of you rise and fall. Feel the breath flowing through you. I want to remind you right there that hidden yet vital breath, that's where *you* are. That's where you find your rest while fully awake. This intentional moment is how we reclaim ourselves from a world that demands more of us and from us. You do not have to wait until Saturday or Sunday like our ancestors long before or until a hard day's work is done. You can rest right here and now.

Get in your body with what I call intuitional stretching. What is this? It is precisely what it sounds like. Listen to your body as you stretch. Where are the places that feel tight and confined? When we enter emotionally tight spaces, we constrict our limbs and bodies, creating more stress and anxiety and less time spent in a restful state. Step away if you must in moments like these. Begin with your shoulders and then your arms and allow your body to tell you where to bend or extend next. When we make rest a practice, breathing and stretching bring us back into our bodies. Why is this important? Because our bodies and humanness is the primary thing that feels pocketed when othered.

RECLAMATION: REST AS YOUR BIRTHRIGHT

Often, when we return home and pull back the covers on our bed, perhaps just as Breonna Taylor did, we sleep but rarely do we rest. Our bodies may remember the violence witnessed, the stolen peace; the rest may feel unearned, a privilege not granted. When we sit down on our sofa to unwind like Botham Jean, fear may be present. It is the historical collective and the personal trauma colliding. Because for the Black body . . . the woman body . . . the gay body . . . the trans body . . . the large body . . . for the othered body, resting is different. Even while sleeping, we are alert from the day, the weeks, the years experienced within these bodies of ours. Hearing about Breonna Taylor caused me to question my own notion of freedom. As mentioned earlier, our rest is tied to our liberation. Freedom can feel like rest as opposed to sleep, it is the knowledge that when I close my eyes I am safe and may reclaim the peace that is mine.

When you awake in the morning, ask yourself, do you feel rested and restored? Or do you feel just as depleted as you were the day before? The quality of your rest matters.

Rest is your birthright. Creating practices around rest is one of the many ways you can begin obtaining rest instead of just sleep. First, examine your current bedtime or rest ritual. Do you typically fall asleep with the phone or laptop just inches away? Is the light still on when you awake due to trying to work through the night? Have you separated your workspace from your sleep space in some way before turning in? Look at what is and is not working for you when it comes to how you practice rest.

After doing so, it's time to create a new rest (or bedtime) routine. As a doula, I often have conversations with parents around sleep training within my scope of practice. Sleep training means that parents will put together a plan of sleep for their little ones to begin training them for sleeping through the night. I like to take this same rule of thought for us adults. We, too, need to practice a bit of sleep training, or what I like to call rest training.

So, what does that look like? For us, it looks like diving into what makes us feel safe and supported while sleeping or in leisure. Here are a few of my favorite ways we adults can "rest train":

- Turn down your bed before starting your ritual. A good turndown service produces visual cues that it's time for our nervous system to begin decompressing and winding down.

- Put on a pair of cozy pajamas or that old T-shirt that makes you feel good and takes you back to a place of home. Intentionally putting on night clothes before bed does wonders for our brain by telling it that it's time to settle down for the night. Our nervous system thrives off routines and patterns.

- If you are into skin care, lean into that. If oiling your body or your partner's body feels good, do that. Try giving yourself a hand or foot massage before bed. The practice of self-touch releases serotonin, easing feelings of anxiety and activation.

- Leave your cellphone outside your bedroom door. Think of your bedroom as a sacred space of rest. Often, our cellphones are directly connected to our work and stimulate that place within us to perform. As we enter rest, we throw work and performance out the window (or at least out our bedroom door).

- Set a bedtime. However, if doing so creates anxiety as the time approaches, pay attention to your body, and begin your bedtime ritual when you feel your body becoming sleepy and asking for rest. Listen to your body, and give it what it needs.

- Prioritize a magnesium bath a couple of times a week. Pour a medicinal amount of Epsom salt into your tub. I like to use around 4 to 6 cups. Epsom salt baths can serve as an excellent resource for soothing the tension and pressures of the day. Afterward, rub lavender or Roman chamomile on the bottoms of your feet and the back of your neck.

- Use meditation and prayer as a form of daily rest. The act of relinquishing and releasing the load from your shoulders is a form of speaking and tending to dry bones so that we can continue. Meditating, deepening, and connecting to our breath can also prove to be helpful. Deep breathing for a count of five . . . holding for a count of five . . . and then releasing for a count of five, or what I like to call breathing in circles, is a perfect tool during meditation.

You do not have to earn your rest. I think of my great-great-grandmother Sally, Mama Dear's mother, who worked the fields, dragging her weary body home after a long day in the hot Alabama sun. I think of my great-grandmother Mama Dear, who vowed that her children would never have to work the fields and that they would know the feeling of rest. How she dreamed that her children and their children wouldn't have to take rest as they could find it, but that they could practice it intentionally as their own. I ask that you take a nap, just because. Working your way through depletion has never made anyone better. However, rest has.

Before the crop grows, it begins as a seed resting in the dirt. By resting, we honor our mothers and fathers, whose work and rest were regulated. I rest for my overworked ancestors, who toiled over the land each day until the day they died. I rest for my great-grandmother Alma Williams, who threw a man out of her home for soliciting her children to work his fields. She worked those same fields so that her children would never have to and so that they could experience rest on this side of heaven, her hands dirt-stained as she tucked the seed into its dark soil's bed, obtaining the rest that she would never know. Whom do you honor with your rest?

Journal Prompts

- Where did you inherit your beliefs around rest?
- Identify the beliefs around rest that you are unlearning.
- Whom will you honor with your rest?
- Create your own rest affirmations.

CHAPTER FOURTEEN

Freedom and the Myth of Perfection

The palm tree stands tall and brave. It weathers hurricanes in tropical climates. Some species can grow to be over two hundred feet. Narrow and grand. The date palm and coconut palm. Fruit producing. Many variants of the palm exist in many plant-loving homes, nestled by a bright window. Spiky leaves that stretch high up into the air, defiant of gravity and all of its laws. Have you ever heard the sound of palm leaves rustling in the wind? Here in California, when the Santa Ana winds begin to blow, you can listen to the sound of the palm's leaves shushing, as if they were about to tell a secret or calm a brewing storm.

The palm is not native to North America. The palm we are familiar with here in the U.S. has had to adapt and thrive in a space to which it is not accustomed. It has had to survive and persevere through elements that are not sustainable to growth, let alone natural selection. Yet it grows and continues to bear fruit.

Much like the palm, POC and other marginalized groups are resilient. We've had no choice but to be. Despite four hundred plus years of slavery, oppression, and systemic racism, Black folks are still here. We have had to adapt, reacclimate, and bloom in spaces that were anything but conducive for our growth for survival purposes. This necessary survival is perhaps the primary reason that the question of how I would like to show up never crossed my mind.

"How do you want to show up in the world?" This question was asked by the healer and yogi Koya Webb while facilitating a sound bath. We at her gathering were majority Black and woman. The session was held via Zoom, as we were steeped deep within the global pandemic of 2020, and the outside was an unsafe and volatile place. I sat in my room, lights off at first, allowing the setting sun to appear through my drawn curtains. Eventually the sun faded beneath the horizon, darkening the sky and my bedroom. I sat there with the others in front of our screens in the dark and in a symphony of singing bowls and reverberating chimes. As I lay on my yoga mat, still, the healer asked, "How do you want to show up?" Up until this point, I had never thought about the want. I had always considered the need. How do I *need to* show up in the world? How do I *have to* show up in the world? The "want" hadn't even entered my sphere.

For many folks who find themselves in the "other" category, how we would "like" to show up has never been presented as an option for navigating this world. I had shown up as a partner and mother, the latter being a non-negotiable role. I had to show for my birth clients while navigating a pandemic. I had to show up within my day-to-day work as one of two Black people within a company. Like many, I was also inundated with fear of disappointment and how others would perceive my showing up.

However, a considerable part of thriving is asking this very question and holding the wisdom within our being that we have a say in the matter. When I think of our ancestors' wildest dreams, I like to believe that they had us in mind and that they envisioned a world where I was free not only in body, but in mind and spirit. A massive part of our freedom is our holistic autonomy and its exploration. When I began to look into the question that the healer proposed, I was forced to examine the prioritization of my feelings, mental health, and overall emotional safety.

Top athletes are often asked to show up, in their bodies, and perform. There are athletes who are asked to be present, to cast away the day's real-life experiences and act as if nothing is happening in their world. Often our world would prefer that these modern-day gladiators sacrifice their mental health for the cause of achieving a goal. How fast can you run despite the day that you are having? How many points can you put on the board, although you just experienced massive loss, and now a reporter is asking you about it on national television?

As mentioned in the previous chapter, existing as a minority in a majority environment can leave many activated. Pairing this activation with already present anxiety can lead to internal burnout, extinguishing the light within. I've heard this burnout compared to a teakettle. The teakettle begins with a slow simmer and then gradually builds to a slow and steady bubble, eventually culminating with a whistle, letting the preparer know that it has reached its point of capacity.

How we take in the outside world is no different. We possess signs of simmering within our thoughts that eventually lead to bubbling and unsaid activation, and if we do not pay close attention, eventually the whistle, alerting all that surrounds us that we have reached our point of capacity, sounds off. Sometimes this whistling sounds like panic and isolation, and occasionally like depression and despair. I've read that anxiety looks different in Black women. Sometimes it looks like irritability and unspoken frustration. Perhaps guarded tears that never make the acquaintance of our cheek. When you've seldom experienced the safe space to unload the burdens of many off your shoulders, the privilege of feeling and expressing anxiety or depression remains precisely that: a privilege. I believe this to be so for many who find themselves in the space of others. Our life experience is built differently, often without cushion or tenderness.

The Myth of Perfection

One of the biggest threats to our emotional safety is perfection. How we hold little to no space or gentleness toward self is one of the many ways oppression is played out. We've all felt it before. You are the first POC, the first gay person, the first disabled body, the first pregnant person, the first parent on the job; you are the first . . . You not only fight the fear of failure, but you feel pressure to do everything right. There are no days off. While working in social media at a significant baby-centered brand, I was the first Black person to step into my role. And although there was never external pressure to overperform, I felt the internal pressure to achieve higher numbers, triple the engagement, and curate more content than those who had come before me. I stepped into my role before the 2020 pandemic and had no idea how I would have to shift and change in the upcoming year. For many companies, 2020 challenged everyone to be fluid like water. We were no different in the company where I lent my voice, expertise, and words.

The year would bring a pandemic that forced many out of work or to work from home. Many were glued to their phones, computers, and hours of screentime, which in turn presented an opportunity to nourish and foster community. However, there was also racial upheaval and protests all around. And while I felt the communal grieving of all that was lost that year, I also had to show up within my work offering advice, writing social media anecdotes, and appearing as a face on the world's camera, the internet, to discuss the benefits of skin-to-skin contact and parenting—all of this while the world is on fire and cops are kneeling on Black folks' necks. If the numbers rose, I felt accomplished. If the numbers fell, I felt as if I had failed and that it was my fault. If there was human error, I believed myself guilty of being human, a weight that I'm sure none of my colleagues considered or were aware of.

This vicious cycle of seeking perfection while othered can only be described as carrying the weight of a company's success on your shoulders. For the record, this level of perfection is absurd, because the attitude of White supremacy exists and the ways by which it has infiltrated our worth is just that, absurd. However, when you are the first, or, in my case, one of three Black folks at a company, the internal dialogue and need for perfection permeate your being in unimaginable ways. The permeation felt like heavy bricks layered upon my subconscious shoulders. The world was a complete and utter shit show, and for many of us, we saw the resemblance to the George Floyds and Breonna Taylors within our uncles, our aunts, and our cousins. While the world flared, many were asked to show up and continue life and business as usual. If not by those around us, the fear was summoned by the internal dialogue of panic at exposing our humanity and casting away our superhero cape.

Many of us who have been othered have an unhealthy relationship with perfection. We have been programmed to believe that we have to be better, do better, and have no room for mediocrity. For the most part, unfortunately, that remains true. However, this way of thinking is binding and does not aid our liberation. We must divorce the idea of perfection and show up within our humanity, knowing that it is enough and worthy of celebration. The need for overperforming and strength when we need to pause is familiar. However, I would challenge you to lean into the truth that you are more than enough and welcome to show up as is in all of your vulnerability and imperfection, and dare I say it, your everyday normalcy. This dismantling falls under what is valuable and beneficial to our longevity. I, too, have felt the pressure to show up and save the day within the space that I occupy, as Black women often do. However, I also need to show up for myself, mother my kids from a healthy margin, and be present for the things that matter most.

So how do we unlearn the need for perfection while achieving excellence? You've guessed it. Unlearning and parenting ourselves with gentleness and parenting our children with that same freedom.

It is remaining aware of how much of ourselves we offer to those around us versus how much we provide to ourselves. Does one outweigh the other? Does it seem out of balance? And if so, it's okay. This acknowledgment is where we can begin to repair and reparent ourselves from the idea that we must work harder despite how it affects our overall health and wellness. You are important. You are vital. *You*, not just what you do or how well you perform. Your spirit, joy, and body are essential to your thriving. And while my goal is not to sound harsh, your job does not care about you. Therefore you must. Take this as your permission to take care. This care looks like boundary setting and time appropriation. You do not have to give and give until you are empty. Perhaps your boundary looks like work ends at five. After this time, you close your laptop and silence your phone notifications.

The grass is soft
Daffodils blowing in the wind
Snow falling from the sky
A kiss from a lover
Some of the best things in life are soft and imperfect.

PARENTING OURSELVES OUT OF PERFECTION

This reparenting has been one of the greatest challenges for me. And it makes sense that it would be. This deprogramming and unlearning you, too, may find difficult and perhaps even impossible. Like grief, this, too, is hard work and heart work, as in this reparenting, there are many things we must let die. In this unlearning of perfection, we are unlearning the programming of our younger selves and parents, our ancestors, and the messaging that their oppressors beat into them. This work goes deep. And let me be clear, this reparenting is not only for those of us whose ancestors were enslaved or from the diaspora. This reparenting is for us all who are other and those in positions of power. Just as I have had to reparent myself out of perfection and its weight, the majority group, White and Man, must also reparent themselves, acknowledging privilege, distancing themselves from colonizer to seeker of equity and equality. Asking themselves, what are the ideas that perhaps continue to serve me but have never served the whole of humanity.

So how do we begin on the road to reparenting and undoing what's already been done? We distinguish the load that's ours to carry from the load that's been unknowingly placed upon us. Remember the passenger thoughts. The idea that we must always be perfect without blemish and that our excellence should only be praised, forsaking our humanness. All of this can be filed under passenger thought. This belief is not ours to carry, but a passenger thought we've picked up on the car ride. Ask, "How has the idea of perfection served me? Has it supported my freedom or created a shackled life?" More than likely, while we can find good moments within our quest for perfection, if we're honest with ourselves, this way of thinking has left us bound and depleted. Why? Because humans are not perfect. You are not the exception to this truth. And when we believe ourselves to be, we bind ourselves to this unrealistic way of living, robbing ourselves of whole-person acceptance and kindness.

Affirm with me: Perfection does not serve me. It shackles me. Today I set myself free.

Another component of reparenting ourselves is radical self-acceptance. All of ourself. All of who we are. I want you to know that you are allowed to have an off day (both calling off from emotional and physical labor, and being emotionally off). So many of us were pushed as kids to be better, to strive through tears, neglecting inner pain. So many of us were taught that our rage is not accepted here, so it remained quiet. And because of this, fear finds its way to the surface, and our authentic self never entirely emerges. We who are othered have versions of ourselves we show to each other like a secret, and then there is the version we offer to others outside our world. We twist and bend and contort our self-expression in the name of assimilation. We closet our queerness and change our speech and familiar tongue. We shrink and make ourselves palatable, hoping not to frighten the opportunity or person away.

In moments like these, I want you to remember the palm tree. Tall and courageous. Although it has adapted to simply survive, it does not assimilate. The palm remains tall and wild in a foreign land now home, refusing to embody the expectations or weight of its environment as its leaves sway with the wind, untroubled and untamed. Maybe this is how we remain carefree while being othered? Your magnificence and standout differences are a sight to behold, not to bury.

Affirm with me: My existence is not too much. My normal is worthy of celebration. My best today is my best. I leave room and kindness for my humanity.

We reparent ourselves out of perfection by genuinely knowing . . . Wait for it . . . We do not have to be good at something to enjoy it. We can even suck! This may sound super simple. However, overthrowing the idea that we must be is not so simple. For example, one of my favorite pastimes is painting with watercolors. Am I good at it? No. You will likely not find my paintings at your local art gallery. I don't even hang them around our home for display. However, I enjoy creating them. I find solace in dipping my dampened brush in the watercolor, spreading it across my canvas, and watching as one color slowly fades into the next. I love how painting slows down my thinking, allowing me to be while trusting my creation's process and myself. It affirms that I can lean into intuition, even in something as simple as watercolor painting.

I want you to know that you can find joy in things you are not good at. I know. We were taught to strive to be the best or at least suitable at the tasks we put our effort into. Otherwise, what's the point? However, I would like to challenge you to dismantle this belief, as it is limiting. It limits us to pursuing only things we can monetize, things we excel at, instead of following our highest joy. Our highest peace. Both are priceless and our most sought entity and treasure. Give yourself room to play. By granting ourselves this freedom, we discover untapped places that we were forbidden by our parents, society, and culture to explore. When we tap into these new and undiscovered joy-filled places, we can create the inner world we want to live in, creating a healthy container to offload the weight of being othered.

Affirm with me: I do not have to be good at something to enjoy it. My joy is reason enough.

RAISING THE NEXT GENERATION OF THRIVERS

"Don't act like that, White people are watching." Chances are if you grew up Black, this phrase has either been said to you or implied by your mother, father, grandmother, grandfather, or some parental figure. I remember growing up with this implied mandate. An idea that I am aiming to break for my children. However, I found myself in this tightrope balance between raising carefree Black kids and kids aware that the rules are not as straightforward as black and white. How do I raise carefree Black kids in a society where Black men, women, and even children are gunned down for attempting to present their license and registration at a traffic stop, for selling cigarettes, for sleeping, for jogging, for being a child? How can I teach them to exist free when I know that the world and this country may view this freedom as a threat? This conundrum is what most people raising children of color find themselves navigating through daily.

Many years ago, when our boys were much younger, we were lying on our blankets in the park. Before I knew it, Jax (my oldest) and Jedi (then my youngest) went in opposite directions to interact with our fellow sunbathers. Jax, then only nine years old, began playing with sticks, stacking them into architectural structures. One-year-old Jedi walked over to a young woman who happened to

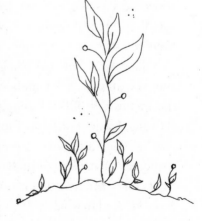

be lying near us and attempted to grab her phone to play. At that moment, I found myself doing something that I knew I'd done before. However, until that moment, I had never questioned why. I began watching. I found myself making sure that my boys were polite, perfect, not too loud, not too rowdy. I wanted to ensure that the slightest childlike move wasn't misinterpreted as aggressive and that the adults watching them felt comfortable. I paused. Why? Why was I uncomfortable? Why was I so afraid? At this moment, I realized that I cared what these White strangers were thinking about my Black sons. Why did I care? The answer hit me, or more so, the question, "How do I raise carefree Black kids who aren't afraid of (and could care less about) the White gaze?"

Where was this fear birthed? Much like an old quilt, this way of thinking was passed down to us by our ancestors. I believe that it came from a place of protection. During the days of my grandmother and great-grandmother, behaving "too free" could get you lynched. In 1955, a fourteen-year-old boy named Emmett Till was beaten, shot, and mutilated for being too free. Fast-forward, and you have Jordan Davis, who was gunned down for being a teenager and playing his music too loud with his friends at a local gas station. In 2014, twelve-year-old Tamir Rice was shot by local police for playing with a toy gun. Truthfully, there are too many to name.

A long list of people lynched, beaten, or gunned down for simply being too Black and or too carefree. Perhaps this is why this unsaid rule of Black people being on their best behavior and showing up in palatable forms has been ingrained into our psyche. Back in the day, it was a matter of life or death. While our country has made much progress from slavery and civil rights days, the question remains: Has this necessary fear truly evolved? And to what degree? No, we no longer see strange fruit hanging from trees. However, Black people being memorialized via hashtags has become the new norm. How do I teach my boys that they matter? How do I teach them that they have every right to feel deeply and express their emotions freely without fear of becoming a hashtag? The answer is twofold. I teach them that their feelings and their social development matter. I teach them that they have the right to express their emotions without fear.

The fearlessness begins at home. I remember the day when Jon and I decided to opt out of the practice of spanking. We both grew up in the South, in the '80s, and with Black parents. And while I grew up not receiving half of the beatings that many folks within my community did, I grew up in a household that believed in the notion of "spare the rod, spoil the child." Like many parents who practiced this form of discipline, I think, within my heart of hearts, they felt they were doing "the right thing." And truthfully, if you look at the origin of this form of punishment and discipline, our parents, grandparents, and great-great-grandparents were doing what they had been taught. Spanking, beating, this was their way of keeping their children safe.

When referring to slavery, physically disciplining your child before Master did so was wise. We at least loved our children, he did not, and his beatings could result in their death. The exact form of discipline continued well past the shackles and chains. As James Baldwin said, "To be Black and conscious in America is to be in a constant state of rage." The same is true regarding parenting while Black. To be a Black parent in America is to be in a constant state of fear. Fear of what the outside world will do to our children if they are not wise beyond their years and blameless. Fear of what happens to cute little Black kids who one day grow into adults, and their cuteness can no longer serve as their protection.

And this fear doesn't cease to exist only for parents of Black children; it exists for any parent of a child that may experience othering. Many of us raising these beautiful children recognize that the world is cold and cruel, and the discipline and safety that we have been taught to distribute for children like ours comes from a place of love, fear, and survival. We want our children to survive the blunt and brash realization that the world doesn't care and that it will devour, feast on, and spit out the cultural bones of the consumed. So what do we do? We try to prevent our children from ever making mistakes and sometimes from being who they indeed are, so they never feel this devastatingly dangerous reality.

Allow me first to say that there is no shame here. As parents, we do what we know and feel to be suitable for our children. And most important, our actions spring forth from a place of love. I refer to physical discipline or spanking as a fear-based parenting method to highlight the root of the action. If we recognize the origin as fear, we can remove shame and humanize our behavior toward our children and show grace to ourselves. If we acknowledge our reason for spanking is fear, we can address the fear, ensuring that we don't project or pass along our worries to our children. After external and internal research, Jon and I decided to opt out of spanking as a form of punishment, as our focus was not punishment but the lesson learned.

Now, I know you may ask, "Why this tidbit on parenting being shared in the section on being othered?" It's because othered kids grow up to be othered adults. It is up to us as their guides to nurture their freedom to flourish and grow up to be fearless adults who thrive in the spaces they occupy. Their first lesson in learning love and self-acceptance is through us, their teachers. The adults.

I remember spanking never really sitting right with me early in my parenting journey. And after the research, realizing why. According to a study by Jorge Cuartas of the Harvard Graduate School of Education, "spanking may alter neural responses to environmental threats in a manner similar to more severe forms of maltreatment." The study was comprised of 147 children. Some experienced spanking as punishment, and others' parents used nonphysical means of discipline. As children were studied via MRI, they were shown images of facial expressions, ranging from smiles to frowns. They found that children who had been spanked possessed a higher brain activity response to a threat even when the facial expressions shown would be considered nonthreatening. These children sensed dangers where there were none. Spanking also has implications for these same children to develop mental health disorders, such as anxiety and depression, as adults. Research shows that spanking creates a chasm within the parent-child relationship and is considered harmful in the long term by the American Academy of Pediatrics.

In the long run, physical punishment, or, as I refer to it, fear-based parenting, doesn't propel our children into reflecting on their decisions and shifting their actions. It puts them into flight, fight, or freeze mode. And when our nervous system is in this state, it is virtually impossible to make decisions, let alone the right ones. Our kids will be adults longer than they will be children. The long goal is to raise adults equipped to make healthy decisions. Not because Mom and Dad will find out and hand down punishment and guilt them into doing the right thing, but because they realize that making healthy decisions creates freedom and will be best for them.

Now, I'm not about to lie. Proceeding in the way of gentle parenting is not easy. It's hard work! And that's not to say the alternative is more effortless. Spanking is just temporarily effective, as there is a possible cost paid later. Attempting to talk a four-year-old through a meltdown is way more complicated and can take a bit longer than immediately popping them on their backside and fearing them into emotionally moving on. However, I would encourage you to consider, what if your four-year-old is melting down merely because they are hungry? You and I have been there before. How often have you acted in a way that you are not proud of because you are hangry or tired? Our children are no different. By taking a breath during these challenging moments and inviting our children to take a moment and focus on their breath, we shift their focus to solutions and internal evaluation. Ask them, "What is it that you need? Are you hungry?" By doing this, we are teaching our children that their feelings, emotions, and bodies matter and just how connected all three are. And we are communicating that we are here to support them while navigating challenging moments like this.

The world may be scary to our children. But our arms and hands should be a safe space. Jon and I both decided that our goal was to raise healthy humans who could thrive in a sea of sharks, not just survive. For us, spanking was not the way. Although tiring, respectful conversations would hopefully produce adults who would know how to navigate their feelings without fear of judgment or shame.

We also wanted our children to feel free to make mistakes. When you are growing up, mistakes are inevitable. However, when you are othered, you are judged most harshly when you misstep. There is a somatic pressure to do everything right—cue perfection, which is another specific tool of oppression. Suppose you do not make mistakes. You don't learn. When you stop learning, you stop growing. When you stop growing, parts of you, the best parts perhaps, die. By allowing the space for our kids to make mistakes and find their way, as we provide guidance, they are learning and soaking in all of the cues around them when they miss it. Substituting curiosity for shame, asking them when they don't choose well, "Well, why did you do that?" Allowing them to answer gives them the gift of reflecting inward.

To raise healthy future adults, we have to ask ourselves from what place we are parenting. Are we parenting from a place of fear? A place of rejection? Are we parenting for acceptance into the Perfect Parents of Perfect Children Awards? If you are parenting from a place of fear, check it. Unchecked fear becomes unchecked reactions as opposed to responses. Ask, "Where is this coming from? What part of me is activated?" Once we identify the source of the fear—the fear of the treatment of the outside world, perhaps?—know that you can combat this fear with love. Fearless and inquisitive kids become bold and curious adults. And these kinds of adults change the world, showing up as they want.

This advice also applies to the nature of reparenting our adult selves. By reparenting using this model of not beating ourselves up when we misstep and shedding the fear of perfection, we are setting ourselves on the path of showing up as we like in this world. Every time we nurture our inner child and ask, "Now why are you feeling this way? What do you need at this moment to feel safe, settled, and whole?" we replace shame with wonder. Our inner child will answer and speak to us, sharing what is needed for them to show up in the world, if nothing else, happy.

So how do we thrive while being othered? We begin by asking ourselves the same question that the healer asked during the sound bath. How would you like to show up in this world?

When prompted to show up
When navigating this wild and crazy world
Pause.

OTHERING AND THE INNER CHILD

How would you like to show up? We benefit by asking our current adult self and our child self this question. As I mentioned, I carried the life managerial role for as long as I could remember. So my child self just continued this role into my adulthood. During moments of peace, I would find something or someone to manage and keep safe. I would survey the room and make sure that everyone was okay. It was up to me to release my inner child from this role by first recognizing it. Many of us who reside in this space of other often have to develop armor to keep us emotionally and physically safe. While wearing this armor, there is no time to ask the question, let alone be curious about how we want to exist in this world. We are surviving.

What becomes of the inner child when showing up is based on survival? Our inner child may become locked away in the deepest, furthest, most unacquainted parts of our brain. And can I tell you? Your inner child is the best part of you.

However, we silence our inner child as if they are the enemy. We treat them perhaps worse than the "adults in the room," where some of us come from the place of children being better seen than heard. In this case, our inner child is neither seen nor heard but instead cast away. We forget that they are always present with us. And let me tell you, your inner child is the bright and full light that we have always hoped to be. Ask your child self, "What do we want to be when we grow up?" The goal is to become the glorious and realized dreams of that child. Ask, "How does my inner child desire to show up within this space?" Not how they are accustomed to showing up. Ask yourself, "Where are the ignored places? The silenced places?" Perhaps you were known as a good singer, an exceptional student, or a talented athlete as a child, but the other parts of you were ignored, and now you find it challenging to connect with parts of yourself that aren't superhuman or deemed extraordinary. Maybe you were also a great listener? A good friend? A courageous and free spirit who wasn't afraid to try even if you failed? These attributes are also worthy of your witness. How long has it been since you talked to your younger self? Have you told them how proud you are of who they have become and are on the most elementary level? Have you celebrated yourself on the most ordinary of days? This is how we reconnect.

My inner child would like to show up for the joyful parts, the creative elements of my life, celebrating when we both achieve a dream we had so many years ago while lying in our bed. After asking these questions, I recognized that my inner child did not want to continue in the manager role. I heal myself by reassigning her to the joyful positions, casting away bits of the protective armor that I've carried so very far. Then I can take light into every space I occupy—showing up the way I desire.

We thrive by fighting for our inner child to remain and by showing fear the door. Fear, intimidation, feeling that we don't deserve to be in the room, that we must prove we deserve a seat at the table, are reminiscent of invasive and intrusive actions. The emotions of fear invade, shouting unworthiness, breaking and arresting the truth that says you belong. It barges in as if it has ownership, disheveling peace and implanting feelings of inadequacy. And once it is done with you, it leaves you questioning everything along with your merit, qualifications, and value. When this happens, we must be aggressive with fear. Like Mama Dear, who beat the cop silly, we must challenge the fear, demanding that it produce facts.

I share with my clients that when fear invades, they should ask for receipts. Rarely is fear factual. In our moments of fear's invasion, I have found creating a two-column list to be a supportive tool. List all the fears on one side, knowing they are sometimes birthed from a valid place, not conjured. When examining those fears, know that they have an origin. However, the anxiety and thoughts accompanying the fears are not yours. They are just thoughts sounding the alarm of fear's entrance. Then, on the other side, list your facts. List anything and everything that you know to be true within the moment of invasion. The points can either be the antithesis of the fear presented or something as wholly separate and straightforward as "My feet are touching the floor." By seeing the list of facts, one can remind themselves of what is happening instead of what is being felt. Because much like fear, feelings also are not facts!

FEAR	FACT
I am afraid of disappointing those around me.	I am surrounded by people who love and support me.
FEAR	FACT
I am afraid of appearing unqualified.	No one has all the answers. When in doubt, I can research/ask and gain the clarity I need.
FEAR	FACT
There are no safe spaces for me.	I am safe in my body. I have shelter where I can experience safety.
FEAR	FACT
I have to be perfect.	No one is perfect. Mistakes are a learning tool.

We must disarm the lies that fear tells us. We do this by reminding ourselves that we are worthy of good and that this space, this world, is ours. We can rest in it. We can absorb it deep within our marrow. When you hear the sirens of fear coming down your street, I encourage you to journal all the ways that you matter. When self-doubt enters your door, go outside in nature, place your feet in the grass. Feel the grass, knowing that you are not much different from it. You, too, are grounded, supported, and filled with purpose.

CHAPTER FIFTEEN

On Thriving

*T*here once was a farmer who lived in a rural land. They possessed acre upon acre of lush green pastures, filled with robust crops and prosperous fruit trees. People would come from far and wide to experience, witness, and taste their bountiful harvest. The farmer was generous with their vast piece of heaven on earth and all that it afforded and often referred to the land as their own personal Eden.

The farmer was old and far along in years, and their story was one of mystery, as no one within the community knew their background, how they arrived or acquired the land. Much like the acres of land, the farmer had always been there to the townspeople. People would speculate and try their hand at the farmer's story. Some recollections would involve the farmer in a duel to the death against an evil overlord to acquire the land. Other accounts were much more straightforward, saying that the farmer came from money. The farmer was both an enigma and a myth. However, the people loved them and their generosity to the public.

The farmer didn't have a family and had never married. The farmer enjoyed their life as one. However, the time had come where they felt the need to retire and perhaps begin training someone to take on the farm's responsibilities long after they were gone. So the farmer put an ad in the town paper, announcing their retirement and asking for all to come forward who felt that they had what it took to continue the farmer's legacy or at least had a green thumb. People came from far and wide to accept the farmer's challenge and more than likely assume the farm's harvest.

One by one, they stepped forward, introducing themselves. The townspeople listed their accomplishments, expertise, and experiences one by one, trying to impress the farmer. After weeks of sifting through prospects, the farmer could finally narrow the auditioners to just three people. The three people all presented as different, possessing diverse backgrounds. One of them was an old banker looking for a different life. The other was a mother who had several children back at home. Then an orphaned child who couldn't have been more than twelve years old.

The tests began. The farmer presented to the new acquaintances a farm tool that none of them had ever seen before. It looked like a cross between giant scissors and a rake—the farmer designed this particular tool for pruning and gathering crops together. However, the farmer did not disclose the purpose of the instrument. Instead, the farmer handed it in turn to the banker, the mother, and the orphan and asked them to work with it. One by one, the three people examined the farm tool and one another, attempting to gather hints regarding the mysterious device. The mother glanced over at the young child, as rumor had it that he had worked on a farm with his family before being orphaned.

The child shrugged and began playing a game, hopping over the farm tool. He said that it reminded him of a long pole that he and his family would play a game of hop over. The device convinced the child that it was a much-needed break that the farmer had offered for their enjoyment, rest, and reprieve. The child and mother glanced over at the banker. The tool visibly agitated him. He sat in the corner shaking with fear. His fear turned to anger as he began to assume that the farmer perhaps knew his story. After all, this was a small town. The banker thought everyone knew his brother had been killed in a fight with scissors that looked similar to the tool provided. There was horror in the banker's eyes. Indeed, this tool was a weapon, and he was afraid. He began bracing himself for what was next. The mother gently assured him that although she, too, was unsure of the tool's purpose, this tool was no weapon. The mother gently placed her hand on the banker's head, reassuring him that the farmer couldn't have known and that this was simply an honest mistake. The mother knew that it was for collecting the harvest. In her experience, she would pick her modest crops from her garden with a tool that looked slightly similar. It wasn't the same, but it appeared so, so she began gathering the ready-to-pick crops.

For the mother, the farmer's tool was for harvesting.

For the banker, a weapon.

And to the child, a memory of fun.

Next, the farmer asked the three to gather water for the crops. Without hesitation, they agreed, asking for vessels for watering. The farmer explained that they would have to find the water, so away they went. As they came to a robust brook, the group paused. The banker immediately began filling his container with water. According to his experience, this was as good as it would get. He saw an opportunity. The child immediately jumped in. He remembered the hot summer days of his family jumping in the nearby brook. To him, creeks were for jumping in and enjoying, not for work.

Meanwhile, the mother paused. She fell to her knees as she saw the stillness of the brook. She planted her hands down in the grassy knoll beside the moving waters. She remembered getting baptized in this same brook. She recalled the preacher calling her to the water and angelic voices singing hymns of being brand-new. Tears streamed down her face like the river in front of her. For the mother, the stream was spiritual. It was holy.

Recognizing the sacrament of the moment, the child found his way to land and out of the water. The banker sat near the mother in awe. As she shared her story of finding refuge and salvation in the water, the boy and the banker began to notice the ebb and flow, the rhythm of the blessed stream, how it flowed as if someone or something were controlling its movement, providing it as a proclamation of peace. The three sat along the riverbank, observing its waves. Because of the mother, the brook had now become holy to both the banker and the orphan.

Last, the farmer presented soil to the three. As before, he gave no instructions and simply left the mother, the banker, and the orphan to figure it out. Sure, they had planted their share of gardens. However, this was a farm producing multiple harvests. The mother began digging and shoveling dirt. It was second nature and instinctual. For her, the soil symbolized renewal and growth. Farming would open a fresh start for her and her children. Tears of joy streamed down her face as she imagined the glory of land ownership and the provision it would offer. For the banker, he was a bit disgusted by the earthworms and the smell of manure. However, he persevered. He was over the life that banking presented. He dreamed of relishing in a life of slowing down and enjoying the micromovements that this great earth so often offered, although we are often so unaware of them.

The child grew somber as he studied the dirt. The cadenced shoveling of the soil reminded him of the death and burial of his parents. The very act of planting and placing a thing within the ground conjured memories of his parents no longer being present on the earth. For the orphan, the dirt represented death. The boy's feeling of grief made its way to the surface as he let out a loud and pain-filled cry. The scooping and the shoveling of the dirt took him back to the place of loss and saying goodbye to his beloved mother and father. Before arriving at the farm, he had escaped hardship upon hardship, abuse after abuse, and had hoped to find a new home here on the farm. The old banker held the boy in his arms. The mother held the banker and the boy's hands as they rocked and swayed, similar to the brook previously witnessed. Finally, the two gathered around the young child, gathering his tears within their hands and planting them, too, in the soil.

The farmer returned and gathered the banker, the mother, and the orphaned child together. The farmer had decided to whom to leave the farm. They explained the day-to-day task of farming and its responsibilities to ensure that the crops planted would thrive. The farmer also shared a secret. The secret is that they had been watching and observing the three applicants the entire time. They saw the banker's anger and fear of the mysterious garden tool, the mother's awe of the riverbank, and even the orphan child's tears and grief triggered by the digging of soil. All of which both broke and expanded the farmer's heart. However, what affected the farmer's decision most was how the group considered that each task, the watering of the crops, planting of soil, even the unknown garden tool, represented something different. The farm tool was a moment of play for the child, but it was a weapon for the banker, triggering moments of hurt. And how for the mother, the river was holy and a place of awe, while for the banker, it was simply a resource for watering crops. The farmer said, "For any living thing to thrive, we must acknowledge one another's perspective." To one person, the soil is just soil, dirt to place over the seed for growing and watering. For another, much like the orphaned child, the same earth can also represent death and mourning, unearthing memories too painful to hold, let alone bury.

The farmer announced with great pride that he would be giving his garden of Eden to all three of them, the mother, the banker, and the orphaned child. The way the three were able to consider and see one another's experiences as no less valuable and no less valid than their own was necessary for the continued thriving of the beautiful ecosystem.

The farmer was an orphan whose mother and father had passed away—their mother during childbirth and father who later succumbed to the grief. After living with strangers and distant relatives, the young farmer had decided to leave and set out on an adventure for a better land when they were thirteen. They searched desperately for feelings of home. They would sleep in abandoned warehouses and barns after families had fallen asleep at night, peering into the windows, hoping that one day they would find safety within their surroundings as these families had.

One morning, after wandering and attempting to find a place to sleep, the young farmer overslept. The night before, they had found a quiet and calm place by a brook, laying their head upon a rock, covering themself with the one blanket stuffed into a bag while leaving what was home. This particular night they slept beneath the stars as the sound of the nearby stream lulled them to sleep. In the morning, they were awakened by a gentle hand. The young farmer opened their eyes with a jolt. Standing there was a woman. She was tall with skin the color of the deepest chocolate. Her hair was gray and piled upon her head in no rhyme or reason. She was dressed in a plaid smock that was cinched in the waist, showing the dirt stains on her dress. She clearly worked the land, as the earth was present on her. This stranger exuded a sense of belonging, acceptance, and grounding, like the earth. She looked at the young boy and said, "Get up. Come home." She didn't inquire about the young farmer's story or how they had found their way to the brook. Instead, she responded as if she already knew the roads the young farmer had traveled and how they had arrived by the riverside and this place called here.

Upon hearing her command, the farmer got up and followed. The woman was a farmer. Much like the banker, she had left her previously fast-paced life in search of something more. She taught the young orphan how to farm, care for the crops, and know which season to plant. She became the farmer's mother. The farmer became her son. Before she passed away, she left them the land.

The farmer saw themself within all three of the prospects. Within the orphan boy, as they were also an orphan. Within the banker, as their mother had also opted to switch paths later on in life, proving that it's never too late to change course. The farmer also profoundly felt the mother sharing her story of finding hope and home by the riverside. They, too, remembered a nearby stream becoming their saving grace, shelter, and rest.

> *Our stories*
> *This flesh and marrow*
> *Our deepest dreams and yet unadorned hopes*
> *In the most primary of our desires and thriving.*
> *At our purest humanity, we are the same and good.*

This truth alone has allowed me to thrive, capture, and encompass joy within this life. In nearing the end of our time together, this is the heart of gentle awareness I want to leave you in your mission of thriving.

During our time together, we talked about thriving in and through grief and our relationship with ourself and each other, all while navigating our mental health and being othered. What is this life? I've heard it asked. Why do we lie down, wake up, toil, or even love? Why do we continue through hardship and what seems like hurt beyond repair?

It's simple—joy and the mastery thereof. Our survival depends on it. It is the sunlight that nourishes us. And it is a critical element in our thriving. If we were plants, our joy would be the daylight, in whose glow we all have the right to bask.

Affirm with me: I have a right to joy. It is mine.

I knew I was on a path to thriving when I uttered words I had never thought I'd whisper. Out loud. For all but most importantly (myself) to hear. I said it first without thinking. "I love my life" poured out of my mouth. I paused, almost stunned by my words, and repeated it. "I *love* my life." And then again, this time intentionally: *"I love my life."*

How can this be? How is it that, as humans, we can experience heartbreak and trauma and yet arrive at a place like this? Part of me would like to say resilience or strength. Like the handful of plants that I thought were dead and without life, we, too, live, persevere, and grow. Life itself is fragile; our spirit and will, not so much.

Fortes fortuna adiuvat. Fortune favors the brave. This bravery is our deepest desire to keep going, waking, toiling, and, yes, loving those around us again and again, even in the face of fear and human disappointment. Our spirits are not easily broken, although we appear wilted. I get it. At this moment, you may not be sure if you will ever get here, let alone without thought, will ever carelessly say the words "I love my life." I said them. And

I meant them. And I pray that you, too, no matter what dark places you've touched, get to say these words without thought.

THE STUDY OF KINDNESS AND OUR THRIVING

What's so funny is that I wasn't necessarily experiencing anything profound or breathtaking when I said these words. It was an ordinary Tuesday at a typical farmers market on a stereotypical fair-weathered California day. I'd put Jupiter, my youngest son, in his car seat, strapping him in securely as I had done a million times before. I got in my car, placed my haul of vegetables in the front seat, and sat there, glancing over into the market, when I saw two Black boys walking by. They couldn't have been more than twelve and thirteen years old. They approached the market, hands enclosed by the pockets of their denim pants. They first visited a booth where they collected food vouchers and where I'd seen two older women visiting before so they could receive free fruits and vegetables. Here in California, farmers markets and vendors pride themselves on food equity for all. So it wasn't unusual to see local shoppers young and old, rich and poor, and from all walks of life shopping for their weekly vegetable bounty. As the two boys left the booth, an older bearded gentleman working the market, a honey vendor and beekeeper, reached within his overflow and offered the two boys honey sticks. They took them, said "Thank you," and went on their way. And this was it. This moment made me utter, "I love my life." Nothing special or profound. Just the witnessing of kindness.

Did you know that a study was done on kindness and its over-all effects on our health? Yes, the practice of kindness or living a life of valuing both ourselves and others, giving and acting in service, has been shown to release oxytocin (the love hormone) and serotonin (the satisfaction hormone) and to lower cortisol (stress hormone) levels. All of these benefits increase one's life span, lower blood pressure, and have been shown to support immune health as well as heart health. Are you feeling guarded? Kindness has been shown to open your heart.

Whether you are the giver, receiver, or, as I was, an observer of it, kindness is the key to joy. There I sat in my car, overwhelmed by the simple offering of kindness from the bearded man. Yes, how kind of the farmer to offer something as simple as a honey stick. And also how kind of the universe that I get to have a front row seat to kindness on an ordinary Tuesday. And this witness is not few and far between, but rarely finding itself front and center within my day-to-day. Kindness (even just the witnessing of it) caused me to see the whole picture surrounding my car, my life, and our lives on this side of heaven.

How kind that although this is not everyone's story, it is mine. How kind that despite calloused moments, fear, and heartache, in this moment, in this chapter, our present story, how kind that we, no matter how bright or murky our life has been, get to experience a new day, a continued life. How kind, right? How kind that I get to experience a place like Pasadena, lush with greenery, tree equity, and food equity. How kind that I live in an area where young Black boys are safe and offered honey sticks as opposed to racial trauma. Witnessing kindness (toward others) caused me to relish my own life. And that appreciation and gratitude are a part of our thriving.

Bearing witness to kindness in a world that says there is none is revolutionary, profound, and a practice. Do you know how people go people-watching? In cultivating joy and filling up your cup, I encourage you to go kindness-watching. Intentionally search for it so that you, too, can witness and encounter your version of what I had the honor of experiencing. Our world shows us trauma, pain, and suffering daily on our news channels and social feeds. And many of us consume it without thought. We must actively pursue kindness, so we can remember that with this breath and life that flow through us, at our most human level, we humans are okay. I dare you to go out and search for it. Kindness-watch, if you will. I promise that it will do for you what it did for me. It provided a deep gratitude for the kindness of all the hands that have kept us here and, as the old folks in church said, "saw ahead and provided."

COMPASSION

"Love and compassion are necessities, not luxuries. Without them, humanity cannot survive," said His Holiness the Dalai Lama. And we most certainly cannot thrive without it. In earlier chapters, I spoke about love in all forms—self-love and love for those around us. Love and compassion toward ourselves are how we can navigate life. It connects us, equipping humans to survive a bitter and brutal world. Forgiving each other for our shortcomings and self-erected idols within love's temple and forgiving ourselves for what we now know but didn't then are all steps toward and in the practice of a life of joy. We thrive by showing the same dose of compassion toward ourselves that we extend to others. Joy (nor the way forward) is not found through self-flogging but in our radical acceptance of where we were then and where we are now. This cognitive rebirth is where joy turns our worst hour into our most brilliant day. And the greatest of these is love.

JOY

Joy is cultivated within itself and within discomfort. Joy is a funny friend that loves us something fierce and is found at times on the other side of what feels like her distant sister, discomfort. Have you recognized her after visiting the depths of grief and loss? Maybe you've found her in challenging moments. Our companion joy is not the absence of discomfort. Nor is the reverse the case either. They can exist together even though they feel worlds apart.

Imagine a mountain-filled hike. Your muscles and ligaments are sore, tight, and rigid at times. It's been a while since you've been on this hiking experience. But today, you journey through, touching the leaves of the trees as you venture around. Your feet kick up the dust of the dirt path forward. One foot in front of the other. The goal is the mountaintop. Clouds above cheer you on as you take one step ahead beyond the next. There in that place is discomfort. However, on the other side of this discomfort, perhaps within it, even as you experience pain, resides the joy of accomplishment or at least fresh air kissing your face in congratulation.

In this life, there will be many rooms, similar to the ones discussed in this book, where we will all find ourselves visitors. At times, discomfort may greet you there. However, joy can be a trusted partner in this place *and* on the other side. When I saw that grief, heartbreak, and the day-to-day blow of othering could not and would not devour me, I could then navigate the complex parts and experience joy. You can too.

We cultivate joy by decentering worry as the catalyst and motivation of our daily goings. I say "Busy, busy we are, and worry, worry we do." We worry about the future and fret over the past, leaving little to no room for our dearest and closest confidante, the present. She's with us always, yet ignored and pushed aside for the more attractive suitor, the future, and most visited, the past. What would happen if we spent most of our time with the present instead of what could be? After all, what is, the here and now, is the only thing we know for sure and what we truly possess.

Two promises I've made to myself in embodying joy and my thriving are:

- I will only make mountains out of hills that have been ver-ified. Or simply put, I will not create crises out of unveri-fied facts—this truth you can carry into relationships and your daily life.
- One step at a time. I do not have to rush through life. I can be *here*.

Sometimes I have dreams in which I am back in school, at the same desk where I sat—surrounded by some of the same people from my childhood years. Sometimes not. And often, when in this dream-filled classroom, I am there to learn a lesson. And so I listen. This time, I visited the classroom sitting at the same desk. But this time, I was surrounded by nameless faces. I sat in my wooden seat as the faceless teacher began to speak. They said, "It's not them. It's you. It's always been you. You as the cap-tain." It proceeded in a warm yet authoritative voice as a teacher would, continuing, "Cease abandoning yourself for the peace of others." I awoke hearing the faceless teacher loud and clear. And I hope you do too. It's you. It's always been you. You as the cap-tain of your unbridled thriving. No matter the room or space we occupy, we have always been our heroes, our farmers, tending our way past weeds and watering ourselves past dry earth.

Thriving—although it may look different for each of us, we are all reaching for the same elements. I believe that whatever land we find ourselves temporarily planted in, whether in the shit of grief or on our mountaintop, we have it in us to gather the life, joy, and peace we desire. Your life is here for you to create divine moments in the ordinary. You are here to start anew and grow even when others propose that you be destroyed and scorched by the heat wave of grief. We humans are just that kind of alchemist magic. We can reimagine and reconfirm and re-claim what is ours for the taking. Like the orphan, the banker, and the mother, we all find a way to obtain a place where we are safe and thriving. Home.

Go kindness-watching
Draw a bath of compassion
for yourself and others.
This is how we nurture joy . . .
How we thrive.

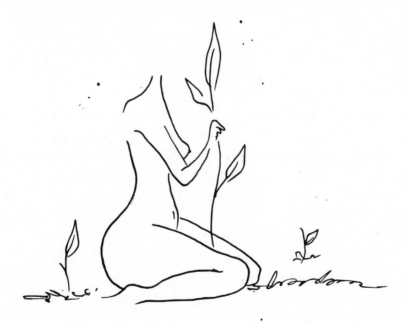

ACKNOWLEDGMENTS

···

Sharing my story has been one of the most profound honors I have ever experienced. This book required that I go back and visit the parts of myself I had long buried away *and* the details that still linger along the surface. In this process, I have many to thank.

I want to thank my wonderful family. Jon, thank you for working to heal and rebuild for yourself first, our children, us all. Thank you for giving me space to tell my story in all its fullness and truth. Thank you for the continued bowls of fancy oatmeal and the reminders that I was more than worthy of sharing my story and its necessity for those who read it. Thank you for keeping the boys occupied and happy so Mommy could write. You did this all during a global pandemic. I could not have done this without you.

Thank you, Jax, Jedi, and Jupiter, my sons, for not always knowing what Mommy was working on in her room but encouraging me to keep going. Thank you for celebrating as if it were your accomplishment when I finally finished writing. Your joy and love are contagious. When you are ready to read this book, I hope you can understand me even more profoundly as your mother and as a co-human who loved you something fiercely, and that there was a beautiful journey to the person you know as Mom.

Thank you, Angela Williams. Thank you for being a constant in my life. Thank you for repeatedly answering late-night calls and meeting me in my grief. While the void of my mother will never be filled, thank you for being as proud when I embarked on this book journey. Thank you for simply showing up and being present.

I want to thank my grandmother, Juril Logan, who showed me as a child what home could be. Thank you for being a safe space and sanctuary. Thank you for allowing me to sit at your feet (virtually) and listen as you shared the story of Mama Dear, your father, Frank Williams, and those who are now ancestors— an experience I will never forget. A special thank-you to Deun Ivory for creating such beautiful illustrations. A huge thank-you to cover director Robbin Schiff for creating this stunning book cover.

Thank you, Meg Thompson, my literary agent, for reading my words and knowing this book was needed out in the world. Thank you for your support, ease, and vision of simply seeing me and knowing what is possible. Thank you for consistently being a guide and North Star for the way forward. I could not have done this without you!

I thank my excellent editor, Chelcee Johns; Sydney Collins; and my Ballantine/Penguin Random House family. I would only want to write this book with you. Chelcee, when we entered this adventure together, you promised to be my word doula. And you have been exactly that. Thank you for pushing me past discomfort and into even more vulnerability. When I was confident I could not go any deeper, you were there to ask the hard questions and push me to discover more. Thank you.

ABOUT THE AUTHOR

BRANDI SELLERZ-JACKSON is a storyteller, birth and postpartum doula, and the creator of *Not So Private Parts*. Initially created as a women's lifestyle blog, *Not So Private Parts* has evolved into a resource removing the shame and stigma surrounding women's issues. Sellerz-Jackson is the co-founder of Moms in Color, a Black mom collective centered on celebrating diversity within the motherhood space. She is also the senior manager of social media at Ergobaby, a leading brand in babywearing and attachment parenting. Brandi Sellerz-Jackson lives with her husband, Jon; their three boys, Jax, Jedi, and Jupiter; and their labradoodle, Chaka, in Pasadena, California.

Instagram: @bstereo

ABOUT THE TYPE

This book was set in Caledonia, a typeface designed in 1939 by W. A. Dwiggins (1880–1956) for the Merganthaler Linotype Company. Its name is the ancient Roman term for Scotland, because the face was intended to have a Scottish-Roman flavor. Caledonia is considered to be a well-proportioned, businesslike face with little contrast between its thick and thin lines.